Nutritional Bioavailability of Iron

Nutritional Bioavailability of Iron

Constance Kies, EDITOR
University of Nebraska

Sponsored by the
Nutrition Subdivision
of the Division
of Agricultural and Food Chemistry
of the American Chemical Society.

ACS SYMPOSIUM SERIES 203

AMERICAN CHEMICAL SOCIETY
WASHINGTON, D. C. 1982

Library of Congress Cataloging in Publication Data

Nutritional bioavailability of iron.
(ACS symposium series, ISSN 0097-6156; 203)

Papers presented at a symposium held at the American Chemical Society meeting in Atlanta, Ga., on Mar. 29–Apr. 3, 1981.
Includes bibliographies and index.

1. Iron—Metabolism—Congresses. 2. Iron in the body—Congresses.
I. Kies, Constance, 1933– . II. American Chemical Society. Nutrition Subdivision. III. Series. [DNLM: 1. Biological availability—Congresses. 2. Iron—Analysis—Congresses. 3. Nutrition—Congresses. 4. Iron—Metabolism—Congresses. QV 183 N976 1981]

QP535.F4N8 1982 612'.3924 82-16391
ISBN 0-8412-0746-1 ACSMC8 203 1-205 1982

PRINTED IN THE UNITED STATES OF AMERICA

ACS Symposium Series

M. Joan Comstock, *Series Editor*

FOREWORD

The ACS SYMPOSIUM SERIES was founded in 1974 to provide a medium for publishing symposia quickly in book form. The format of the Series parallels that of the continuing ADVANCES IN CHEMISTRY SERIES except that in order to save time the papers are not typeset but are reproduced as they are submitted by the authors in camera-ready form. Papers are reviewed under the supervision of the Editors with the assistance of the Series Advisory Board and are selected to maintain the integrity of the symposia; however, verbatim reproductions of previously published papers are not accepted. Both reviews and reports of research are acceptable since symposia may embrace both types of presentation.

CONTENTS

PREFACE

IF NUTRIENTS FOUND IN FOOD were digested, absorbed, and made available to the human or animal body at the 100% level, the science and practice of nutrition would be indeed simplified. That nutrients vary in their bioavailability has been well established. The chemical nature of the specific form of the nutrient involved, the chemical and physical characteristics of the foods in which nutrients are contained, other constituents of the diet, the nature of the digestive and absorptive processes for the specific nutrients, and the physiological condition of the person consuming the food all may affect bioavailability. However, knowledge of specific individual and interacting factors affecting bioavailability and utilization of nutrients has not yet been fully elucidated and constitutes one of the most active areas of current nutrition research.

Iron deficiency anemia is commonly found in both affluent and economically deprived populations. In prevention of this nutritional deficiency disease, both increase in dietary iron and increase in the availability of this dietary iron for population groups at risk should be concurrently addressed. This is a problem for which the solution lies primarily not with the medical community but rather with the providers of food in agriculture and food industry.

The chapters were selected to give a broad overview of the topic of bioavailability of iron with special emphasis on topics of concern to food producers.

The editor expresses appreciation to all the contributors and to Donna Hahn, who did much of the organizational work involved in preparation of this volume.

CONSTANCE KIES
University of Nebraska
Lincoln, Nebraska

July 1982

1

Efficiency of Hemoglobin Regeneration as a Method of Assessing Iron Bioavailability in Food Products

ARTHUR W. MAHONEY and DELOY G. HENDRICKS

Utah State University, Colleges of Family Life and Agriculture, Department of Nutrition and Food Sciences, Logan, UT 84322

The bioavailability of iron from any source (e.g., iron supplement, food or meal composite) is considered to be that portion of the total iron which is metabolizable. Philosophically, this concept is important because the amount of iron utilized by avian and mammalian species is directly associated with iron need. When assaying iron bioavailability, it is therefore necessary to use an organism whose need will exceed the amount provided. In animal assays of iron bioavailability, iron need is assured by a growth phase and/or creation of iron deficiency through feeding an iron deficient diet and phlebotomy. Because healthy subjects are usually used in human assays of iron bioavailability (Cook et al., 1981; Cook and Monson, 1976; Radhakrishman and Sivaprasad, 1980), it is inappropriate to compare the data obtained from animal and human assays. In fact it is questionable if assays of iron bioavailability yield good information on the quantities of metabolizable iron available when healthy human subjects are used.

The Committee on Dietary Allowances, Food and Nutrition Board, National Academy of Sciences (RDA, 1980) has estimated the amount of metabolizable iron (as absorbable iron) from meals consumed by human beings as ranging from 3 to 23 percent depending on the nature of the meal. For adult women of childbearing age, the committee has assumed that 1.5mg iron is lost daily and that 18mg should be consumed to meet this need. They have therefore assumed that approximately 8.3 percent of the dietary iron will be metabolized. For adult men and women over the age of 51 years, they estimate that 1.0mg iron will be lost daily and recommend that 10mg should be consumed to meet this need to offset only approximately 10 percent of the dietary iron being metabolized by these people. It should be noted, however, that what is metabolized from a food under such conditions does not necessarily reflect what is <u>potentially</u> metabolizable. Indeed, the majority of women of childbearing age consume less than the recommended 18mg iron

0097-6156/82/0203-0001$06.00/0

and yet are not iron deficient (DHEW, 1968-70). Thus, much information is needed on the metabolizability of food iron.

Two basic methods have been used in the assay of iron bioavailability (Bing, 1972; Thompson and Raven, 1959). In the absolute method, the change in total body iron relative to that consumed is used. This necessitates making an estimate of the amount of iron present in the animal body at the initiation of the experiment and then determining the amount present at the termination. Usually in applying this procedure, a representative group of animals is killed at the beginning of the experiment to obtain the estimate of their initial body iron. Thus, one can obtain an average value for body iron content relative to weight that can be multiplied with initial body weights to estimate initial amounts of body iron for each test animal. Various modifications of the hemoglobin regeneration procedure have been used(Bing, 1972). In the one described here, the amount of iron gained as hemoglobin is estimated and expressed relative to the amount of iron consumed. An efficiency of the conversion of food iron into hemoglobin can be computed for each test animal knowing initial and final body weights, initial and final hemoglobin concentrations, the amount of food consumed, and the iron content of the food. It is calculated as follows:

$$\text{mg Hb Fe} = \text{BW} \times .067 \text{ ml bl/g BW} \times \text{g Hb/100 ml} \times 3.35\text{mg Fe/g Hb}$$

$$\text{Efficiency} = ((\text{Final mg Hb Fe} - \text{Initial mg Hb Fe}) / \text{mg Fe consumed}) \times 100$$

In applying this method, weanling male rats are given free access to a low-iron diet and bled to remove about one ml of blood two times 4 days apart. Three days later, the animals are again bled of about 100 microliters blood for determination of hemoglobin concentration and are allotted to treatments of ten rats each such that mean body weights and hemoglobin concentrations are similar. The mean hemoglobin concentrations should be between 4 and 6 gm/dl. They are fed the test diets for ten days in amounts that very few orts are obtained. Any spillage and orts are weighed and recorded to account for unconsumed dietary iron. The low-iron diet should contain less than 10 ppm Fe and the test diets should contain approximately 35 ppm. This amount of dietary iron has been shown not to exceed the ability of this animal preparation to utilize iron, since the regeneration of hemoblobin iron is linear at least to 68 ppm dietary iron (Mahoney and Hendricks, 1976). Miller (1977) reported that iron gained as hemoglobin was linear (r=0.94) through intakes of 5.5mg iron as ferrous sulfate in 11 days. Her rats were made anemic by feeding low-iron diet for 24 days in preparation for the hemoglobin regeneration experiment.

The following criteria for a good bioavailability assay are appropriate. (a) It must be dose responsive. For an assay to be useful in a variety of situations, it should not be affected by variations in amounts of iron consumed. Therefore, the dose-response relationship should be linear. (b) It must discriminate with good sensitivity among sources of iron and among treatments such as cooking or processing. (c) Bioavailability values obtained should be unaffected by factors unrelated to the food or iron source. Thus, the bioavailability assay should be insensitive to variations in caloric density of the diet, appetite of the animal, and animal maturity. (d) The procedure should yield reproducible results for the same iron source among experiments and laboratories.

The efficiency of converting dietary ferrous sulfate iron into hemoglobin by anemic rats has been calculated from the data of many experiments and laboratories (Table 1). The 'uncorrected' efficiency values represent the values obtained for the total amounts of iron in the diets and the 'corrected' values represent a mathematical estimation of the hematinic response to only the ferrous sulfate iron present in the diet. This estimate was made assuming that the amount of iron present in the low-iron basal diets reflects the cumulative iron provided by the basal ingredients of the ferrous sulfate test diets (e. g., casein, oil, dextrose, fiber, vitamin mixture and mineral mixture). Thus, knowing the amounts of diet consumed by the test animals, one can estimate the contribution of the basal ingredients to the total dietary intake of iron of the test animals. This value subtracted from the total iron intake yields the estimated iron intake from ferrous sulfate. Similarly, the amount of iron gained as hemoglobin by the rats fed the low-iron basal diet can be calculated and subtracted from the total iron gained as hemoglobin by the rats fed the ferrous sulfate test diets, which yields an estimate of the ferrous sulfate contribution to the iron gained as hemoglobin. This value, relative to the estimated quantity of iron consumed as ferrous sulfate, was used to compute the 'corrected' efficiencies presented in table 1. The 'corrected' values were computed similarly for the iron sources presented in table 2. The validity of this correction is doubtful when foods are the source of experimental iron because the amounts of basal ingredients are decreased depending on the iron content of food tested, which affects the amount of food that must be formulated into the diet to provide the desired iron content.

For ferrous sulfate, the average efficiency of converting dietary iron into hemoglobin was 52 percent with a coefficient of variation of 19 percent (Table 1) . When corrected for the basal dietary ingredients, the average efficiency was 61 percent, with a coefficient of variation of 33 percent. Making the correction for the basal ingredients did not improve the analysis. In two cases, the 'corrected' efficiency of conversion was greater than 100 percent.

Table 1. Efficiency of Converting Iron in $FeSO_4$ into Hemoglobin by Anemic Rats

Dietary Fe (mg/kg)	Efficiency Uncorrected	Efficiency Corrected[a]	Reference
33.0	80	111	Farmer et al. (1977)
40.4	50	52	Allred (1976)
31.2	38	42	Mahoney et al. (1979)
27	71	45	Rahotra et al. (1973)
27	69	44	
--	54	56	Anderson et al. (1972)
27.8	51	70	Mahoney et al. (1974)
16.2	47	68	Blumberg & Arnold (1947)
20.5	48	60	
29.2	52	61	
45.0	46	49	
18.2	44	33	Mahoney & Hendricks (1976)
25.6	41	34	
41.8	46	41	
68.9	36	39	
11.8	57	53	Miller (1977)
18.9	62	60	
23.8	72	71	
23.6	54	42	Cardon et al. (1980)
35.2	60	57	
48.2	66	66	
	49	55	Theur et al. (1971)[b]
	53	59	
	57	62	
	49	50	
	52	85	Theur et al. (1973)[b]
	57	76	
	48	58	
13.8	53	148[c]	Fritz et al. (1974)[b]
19.8	57	89	
31.8	47	61	
12.2	33	39	Fritz et al. (1970)[b]
17.2	38	45	
22.2	43	50	
27.2	42	46	
14	41	58	Shah et al. (1979)
20	60	78	
32	53	60	
15	51	71	Shah and Belonje (1973a)
22	67	81	
32	57	64	
16.5	54	74	Shah and Belonje (1973b)
26.5	57	66	
46.5	43	47	
Mean ± Sd	52 ± 10	61 ± 20	T=2.67 (P .02)

Continued on next page.

Table 1-Continued

Note: Uncorrected efficiencies of 82, 77, 74, 65, 63, 84, 82, and 65 percent were calculated using data presented by Cowan et al. (1967). Because there were insufficient data published to calculate the corrected efficiencies, these data were not included in Table 1.

[a]The efficiency was corrected by estimating the contribution of iron in the basal diet to iron intake and hematinic response.

[b]Supplemental data necessary for computations supplied by authors.

[c]Values greater than 100 percent not included in the mean.

Table 2. Efficiency of Converting Iron From Various Sources Into Hemoglobin By Anemic Rats.

Source	Dietary Fe (mg/kg)	Efficiency Uncorrected	Efficiency Corrected[a]	Reference
$FePO_4$	18.8	26	4	Blumberg & Arnold (1947)
	29.2	18	4	
	54.9	21	18	
	118.0	14	12	
$FePO_4$	19.8	22	34	Fritz et al. (1974)[b]
	31.8	24	32	
	55.8	23	27	
$FePO_4$	24.2	21	26	Mahoney & Hendricks (1976)
	32.6	17	18	
	38.2	23	25	
	49.7	26	30	
Ground Beef	26.6	34	42[c]	Mahoney et al.(1974)
Beef Shank	31.0	63	87	Farmer et al.(1977)
Beef Plate	33.0	61	79	Farmer et al. (1977)
Bologna	29.0	46	62	Mahoney et al. (1979)[b]
Beef	26.0	49	37	Cardon et al. (1980)
Turkey	23.0	45	74	Mahoney et al. (1980)
Turkey	30.4	43	---	Cardon et al. (1980)
Enriched Flour	24.4	24	33	Mahoney et al. (1974)
White Bread	10.7	28	49	Miller (1977)
Whole Wheat Flour	28.0	43	54[c]	Mahoney et al.(1974)
Rice	28.0	30	31	Shah et al. (1979)
	48.0	43	41	
Dried Egg	21.2	43	41	Mahoney et al.(1974)

[a]The efficiency was corrected by estimating the contribution of iron in the basal diet to iron intake and hematinic response.

[b]Supplemental data necessary for computations supplied by authors.

[c]Due to calculation errors, the original value was reported as 45 for ground beef and 33 for whole wheat flour.

In ten cases, the 'corrected' values were less than the uncorrected ones. Because of this inconsistency and because correction does not reduce variability within nor among experiments, attempting to correct for the iron contribution of the basal ingredients to the hematinic response does not seem to improve this assay of iron bioavailability.

Dietary iron level does not seem to affect the efficiency with which dietary iron is converted into hemoglobin when ferrous sulfate (Table 1) or when ferric orthophosphate (Table 2) is the primary source of dietary iron. This is also true for white bread (Table 2); however, the source of the iron in the enriched flour used in the bread is unknown. That the efficiency of converting food iron into hemoglobin is not affected by dietary iron concentration is important to bioavailability testing because it is often difficult to formulate diets with precise amounts of iron, especially when foods are the sources of iron.

The effects of carbohydrate and fat on the efficiency with which dietary iron is converted into hemoglobin have been studied. Miller and Landes (1976) used starch, sucrose or glucose as the carbohydrate source and ferrous sulfate as the iron source. The respective efficiencies of converting dietary iron into hemoglobin were 72, 65, and 46 percent. Amine and Hegsted (1971) obtained similar carbohydrate effects studying iron absorption. Glucose is the most commonly used source of dietary carbohydrate in semipurified diets. Pennell et al. (1976) reported that beta-lactose in place of sucrose reduced the relative biological value of iron as sodium iron pyrophosphate when fed to rats. However, alpha-lactose or glucose in place of the sucrose did not affect the bioavailability of this iron source. Similarly, the source of fat can affect the bioavailability of dietary iron; but, the level of dietary fat has no effect (Mahoney et al., 1980). The casein concentration of diets fed rats does not affect iron absorption (Amine and Hegsted, 1971, Carmichael et al., 1975); however, effect of protein source was not studied by these authors. Thus, the sources of carbohydrate and fat can markedly affect the utilization of dietary iron and should be considered as important variables in bioavailability experiments. The amount of protein, however, does not seem as critical.

Among experiments, the variability of the efficiency of converting iron from ferrous sulfate into hemoglobin (Table 1) was much greater than when ferric orthophosphate (Table 2) was the iron source. This variability is disturbing since ferrous sulfate is commonly used as a reference source of iron for bioavailability experiments, as well as an iron supplement clinically. Typically, this variability is dealt with by expressing the hematinic responses of the unknowns relative to ferrous sulfate (Shah et al., 1979; Coccodrilli et al., 1976; Amine et al., 1972).

Using the efficiency of converting dietary iron into hemoglobin, effects of food processing procedures on the bioavailability of iron in meat have been studied. Farmer et al. (1977) showed that the bioavailability of iron from mechanically deboned meat was less than that from hand deboned meat; but, more metabolizable iron was available in the mechanically deboned product because of its greater iron content. There was no difference, however, between the iron bioavailability from mechanically deboned and hand deboned turkey frame meat (Allred, 1976). The difference in iron bioavailability between the mechanically deboned turkey and the mechanically deboned beef might be attributed to differences in abrasiveness of the meat and bone mixture on the machinery, which would modify the amount and form of iron in the two products (Farmer et al., 1977). The bioavailability of meat iron is decreased due to curing. This decrease is dose dependent with nitrite added, until residual nitrite begins to accumulate (Mahoney et al., 1979). Residual nitrite was associated with an apparent increase in iron bioavailability, which was explained on the basis of some nitric oxide binding to hemoglobin, rendering a fraction of it unable to carry oxygen and thus stimulating hematopoiesis. Severe atmospheric oxidation of beef results in depressed iron bioavailability and growth in rats while similar oxidation of turkey meat did not (Cardon et al., 1980).

Based on the limited data available, the relative biological values of iron sources are similar whether determined by the slope-ratio assay or by efficiency of conversion of dietary iron into hemoglobin (Table 3). The most descrepancies are observed when the relative biological value is estimated by method "c" in Table 3. Much additional research is required to determine the utility of the simpler method of evaluating iron bioavailability by efficiency of converting dietary iron into hemoglobin. It does, however, take less time than the slope-ration method, apply to food stuffs of relatively low iron concentration (Ifon, 1981), provide for direct measurements of iron utilization, and apply to human subjects such as blood donors, anemic subjects (Norby and Solwell, 1977) and infants (Garry, et al., 1981). It, therefore, has many potential advantages as means of evaluating iron bioavailability.

Table 3. Comparison of Biological Values of Different Iron Sources Relative to Ferrous Sulfate

Iron Source	Rel. Biol. Value	Reference
$FePO_4$	51[a]	Mahoney & Hendricks (1976)
$FePO_4$	56[b]	Amine et al. (1972)
$FePO_4$	44.5 ± 4.8[b]	Fritz et al. (1974)
$FePO_4$	23[a]	Blumberg & Arnold (1947a)
$FePO_4$	46[a]	Blumberg & Arnold (1947b)
$FePO_4$	14[c]	Fritz et al. (1970)
$FePO_4$	75[c]	Motzok et al. (1977)
$FePO_4$ in Breakfast Cereal	33[c]	Shah et al. (1979)
$FePO_4$ in Breakfast Cereal	38[c]	Coccodrilli et al. (1976)
Enriched Flour	55[a]	Mahoney et al. (1974)
Enriched Flour	32[c]	Fritz et al. (1970)
White Bread	53[b]	Miller (1977)
Turkey, raw	83[a]	Mahoney et al. (1980)
Turkey, raw	72[a]	Allred (1976)
Whole egg, dried	84[a]	Mahoney et al. (1974)
Egg yolk	33[c]	Fritz et al. (1970)
Beef, raw	80[a]	Cardon et al. (1980)
Beef, cooked	67[a]	Mahoney et al. (1974)

[a]Relative Biological Value calculated by dividing the efficiency of converting iron from the test diets into hemoglobin iron relative to that for diets containing ferrous sulfate.

[b]Relative Biological Value determined by slope-ratio assay.

[c]Relative Biological Value is calculated (Pla and Fritz, 1971):

$$RBV= \frac{\text{mg Fe/kg from test diet}}{\text{mg Fe/kg from } FeSO_4 \text{ diet}} \times 100 \text{ that give the same response in hemoglobin}$$

Acknowledgments

This chapter is Journal Article No. 2681 of the Utah State University Agricultural Experiment Station.

Literature Cited

Allred, L. C. "Some Effects of Mechanical Deboning on the Composition and the Bioavailability of Protein and Iron in Turkey Frame Meat", M.S. Degree Thesis, Utah State University, Logan, Utah (1976).

Allred, L., Mahoney, A. W., Hendricks, D. G. Nutr. Rpts. Intl. 14, 575 (1976).

Amine, E. K., Hegsted, D. M. J. Nutr. 101, 927 (1971).

Amine, E. K., Neff, R., Hegsted, D. M. J. Agr. Food Chem. 20, 246 (1972).

Anderson, T. A., Kim, I., Fomon, S. J. Nutr. Metabol. 14, 355 (1972).

Bing, F. C. J. Am. Dietet. Assoc. 60, 114 (1972).

Blumberg, H., Arnold, A. J. Nutr. 34, 373 (1947a).

Blumberg, H., Arnold, A. Cereal Chem. 24, 303 (1947b).

Cardon, K. M., Anthony, R. J., Hendricks, D. G., Mahoney, A. W. J. Nutr. 110, 567 (1980).

Carmichael, D., Christopher, J., Hegnenauer, J., Saltman, P. Am. J. Clin. Nutr. 28, 487 (1975).

Coccodrilli, G. D., Jr., Reussner, G. H., Thiessen, R., Jr. J. Agr. Food Chem. 24, 351 (1976).

Cook, J. D., Monsen, E. R. Am. J. Clin. Nutr. 29, 859 (1976).

Cook, J. D., Morck, T. A., Lynch, S. R. Am. J. Clin. Nutr. 34, 2622 (1981).

Cowan, J. W., Esfahani, M., Salji, J. P., Nahapetian, A. J. Sci. Fd. Agr. 18, 227 (1967).

Department of Health, Education and Welfare. "Ten-State Nutrition Survey 1968 - 1970", DHEW Publication Nos. (HSM) 72-8132 and (HEM) 72-8133.

Farmer, B. R., Mahoney, A. W., Hendricks, D. G., Gillett, T. A. J. Food Sci. 42, 1630 (1977).

Fritz, J. D., Pla, G. W., Harrison, B. N., Clark, G. A. J.A.O.A.C. 57, 513 (1974).

Fritz, J. C., Pla, G. W., Roberts, R., Boehne, J. W., Hove, E. L. J. Agr. Food Chem. 18, 647 (1970).

Garry, P. J., Owen, G. M., Hooper, E. M., Gilbert, B. A. Pediatr. Res. 15, 822 (1981).

Ifon, E. T. Nutr. Rpts. Intl. 24, 25 (1981).

Mahoney, A. W., Hendricks, D. G., Gillett, T. A., Buck, D. R., Miller, C. G. J. Nutr. 109, 2182 (1979).

Mahoney, A. W., Farmer, B. R., Hendricks, D. G J. Nutr. 110, 1703 (1980).

Mahoney, A. W., Hendricks, D. G. Nutr. Metabol. 20, 222 (1976).

Mahoney, A. W., Van Orden, C. C., Hendricks, D. G. Nutr. Metabol. 17 223 (1974).

Miller, J., Landes, D. R. Nutr. Rpts. Intl. 14, 7 (1976).
Miller, J. J. Agr. Food Chem. 25, 154 (1977).
Motzok, I., Davies, M. I., Verma, R. S. Pennell, M. D. Nutr. Rpts. Intl. 15, 459 (1977).
Norby, A., Solwell, L. Scand. J. Haematol. Suppl. 32, 270 (1977).
NRC/NAS. "Recommended Dietary Allowances", 9th ed., National Academy of Sciences, 2101 Constitution Ave., NW., Washington, D. C. 20418 (1980).
Pennell, M. D., Davies, M. I., Rasper, J., Motzok, I. J. Nutr. 106, 265 (1976).
Pla, G. W., Fritz, J. C. J.A.O.A.C. 54, 13 (1971).
Radhakrishnan, M. R., Saviaprasad, J. J. Agr. Food Chem. 28, 55 (1980).
Ranhotra, G. S., Loewe, R. J., Puyat, L. V. Cereal Chem. 50, 745 (1973).
Shah, B. G., Belonje, B. J. Inst. Can. Sci. Technol. Aliment. 6, 37 (1973b).
Shah, B. G., Belonje, B. Nutr. Rpts. Intl. 7, 151 (1973a).
Shah, B. G., Giroux, A., Belonje, B. J. Agr. Food Chem. 27, 845 (1979).
Theurer, R. C., Kemmerer, K. S. Martin, W. H., Zoumas, B. L., Sarett, H. P., J. Agr. Food Chem. 19, 555 (1971).
Theurer, R. C., Martin, W. H., Wallander, J. F., Sarett, H. P. J. Agr. Food Chem. 21, 482 (1973).
Thompson, A., Raven, A. M. J. Agr. Sci. 52, 177 (1959).

RECEIVED July 30, 1982.

2

In Vitro Estimation of Food Iron Bioavailability

DENNIS D. MILLER and BRIAN R. SCHRICKER

Cornell University, Department of Food Science, Ithaca, NY 14853

A simple, rapid, and inexpensive in vitro method for estimating food iron availability is described. The method involves a simulated gastrointestinal digestion using commercially available enzymes. Soluble, low molecular weight iron is used as an indicator of iron availability. Similar results are obtained when the soluble iron is intrinsic food iron or added extrinsic radioiron. The method is designed to be used with single foods or complex meals. Results obtained with this method compare favorably with published results from human studies using extrinsic radioiron tag methods. The method resembles several published in vitro methods but is unique in two ways: 1. pH adjustment is achieved by dialysis. 2. Low molecular weight soluble iron rather than total soluble iron is used to estimate available iron.

It is well established that evaluation of diets for iron adequacy requires knowledge of both the amount and the availability of the iron present (1). While information on the iron content of foods is reasonably adequate, knowledge of food iron availability is incomplete. This gap in our understanding of the potential of dietary iron to meet nutritional needs exists because a number of complex and interacting factors influence food iron availability and because iron availability is difficult to measure. Iron absorption from a food is affected not only by the chemical form of the iron in the food but also by the iron status of the person consuming the food, the presence of other foods in the same meal, the amount of acid secreted by the stomach, the rate of passage of the food through the digestive tract, and, most likely, other factors. The experience of numerous investigators has shown that accurate measurement of iron availability is a difficult, expensive and time consuming process. The occurrence in the literature of frequently conflicting data attests to

0097-6156/82/0203-0011$06.00/0

the fact that food iron availability measurements are fraught with difficulties.

The objective of this paper is to discuss an in vitro method we have developed for estimating food iron availability. The paper will be presented in three sections: 1. Rationale for the design and utility of an in vitro method. 2. A description of the in vitro method. 3. Results and evaluation of the method.

Rationale

Current methodology for estimation of food iron availability usually involves one of three approaches: animal bioassays, human bioassays, or in vitro measurements.

The most frequently used animal bioassay is the rat hemoglobin repletion test. Fritz, et al. (2), Miller (3), and Rotruck and Luhrsen (4) have described the method in detail. The method depends on the ability of an iron source to increase the hemoglobin concentration in anemic rats. Principal advantages of this method include: 1. the use of an intact biological system, 2. the relative simplicity of the method, and 3. the availability of the method to a large number of researchers. The drawbacks of this method are: 1. the problems associated with the extrapolation of results from rats to humans, 2. the requirement that anemic animals must be used (relative iron availabilities may differ between anemic and nonanemic animals), 3. requirement for graded levels of iron in the diets (when whole foods are used this means that the composition of the diets is usually not constant between groups), and 4. the expense associated with the method.

A second animal bioassay method is the whole body counting method which has been described by Welch and Van Campen (5). In this method, food containing a radioactive tracer is given to the animals in a single dose and retention of the tracer in the whole animal over time is measured. Advantages include: 1. the use of an intact biological system, 2. the simplicity of the method (frequent blood sampling and food consumption measurements are not required), 3. the flexibility of the method (animals in different treatment groups may or may not receive identical diets throughout the experiment, depending on the study design requirements), and 4. the option to use either anemic or nonanemic animals. Disadvantages include: 1. questions regarding extrapolation of results to humans, 2. requirements for specialized equipment (whole body counter), and 3. questions about extent of exchange of tracer and endogeneous iron when an extrinsic label is used.

The most frequently used human bioassay method is the two pool extrinsic radioiron tag method (6). The method is based on two assumptions. One, that food iron exchanges with two common pools in the gut (heme and nonheme iron pools) and two, that added radiolabeled heme iron exchanges completely with food heme iron and added radiolabeled nonheme iron exchanges completely with food nonheme iron. Incorporation of the radioiron tag into hemoglobin is used as the response parameter. This method has proven to be very successful (7). Advantages include: 1. the use of human subjects and, therefore, elimination of questions regarding extrapolation, 2. the simplicity of the method (a single dose containing the radio labeled food is administered and a blood sample is drawn two weeks later for counting). Disadvantages include: 1. the administration of radioisotopes to human subjects, 2. restrictions in the use of the method (relatively few investigators are licensed to administer radioisotopes to human subjects for purely research purposes), and 3. the wide inter-subject variability in iron absorption. (This variability can be largely overcome by using each subject as their own control and by administering a reference dose).

In vitro methods have been used to estimate iron availability for at leat 50 years (8). Two approaches with various modifications have been used. One approach is to measure "ionizable " or "ionic" iron in foods. This is done by determining the fraction of the total iron in a food that will react with a complexing agent such as α,α'-dipyridyl (8) or bathophenanthroline (9) to form a chromagen which can be quantitated spectrophotometrically. A second approach is to subject the food to a simulated gastric or gastrointestinal digestion using purified peptic and/or pancreatic enzymes with subsequent measurement of the soluble iron released by the digestion (10-13). Advantages of in vitro methods include: 1. their low cost and speed, 2. their reduced variability compared to in vivo methods (variability caused by differences in iron status of animals and humans is avoided), and 3. the ability to precisely control conditions during the determinations. Disadvantages include: 1. uncertainties over the use of an artificial system, 2. the less than exact duplication of in vivo conditions, 3. the inability to account for effects of active transport, brush border binding proteins, etc.

It is clear that each approach has its advantages and disadvantages and that all three approaches have provided and will continue to provide information on food iron availability. It is also clear that further development and evaluation of the three approaches will enhance the usefulness of the data generated by them.

Development of conditions suitable for a successful in vitro method requires careful attention to conditions present in the gut during digestion and to the behavior of iron in solution. The environment in the GI tract and the chemical form of the iron both in the food and in the digesta interact to determine the fraction of the food iron that is available for absorption.

The primary determinants of food iron availability are: 1. the extent of iron release from food and 2. the solubility, molecular weight, and stability of complexes formed from the released iron. A large number of factors interact to influence these determinants.

The nonheme iron in food is most likely bound to food components, probably protein. The release of iron from these components is a complex process. It is reasonable to assume that the binding affinity of the food components for iron, the digestibility of the food components, the presence of reductants and accepting ligands, the pH in the GI tract are all factors which influence release of the iron from the food. Binding affinity and digestibility are characteristics of the food and may vary significantly between foods. Reductants and accepting ligands are also largely contributed by the food. Digestion products may act as reductants and/or accepting ligands. Food components such as ascorbate, citrate, and simple sugars may contribute substantially to the release of the iron from food.

Since factors which are characteristics of the food would not differ between in vivo and in vitro situations, the major variables that must be controlled in an in vitro simulation are pH, enzyme concentrations and activities, and digestion times.

The observation that iron absorption is reduced when gastric acid secretion is compromised (14) suggests that gastrointestinal pH does influence food iron availability. The explanation for this appears to be related to the importance of acid for the release of iron from food. Bezwoda et al. (15) measured the capacity to solubilize iron in bread of gastric juice from normal and iron deficient subjects. Gastric juices with pH values above 2 had limited capacity to solubilize bread iron while below pH 2, solubilization of iron increased linearly with decreasing pH. Even though the stabilities of metal complexes in foods are unknown, it is to be expected that low pHs will result in greater release of food iron since metal chelate stabilities decrease with decreasing pH (14). It is apparent, therefore, that pH must be carefully controlled in any in vitro method designed to estimate food iron availability. Selection of an appropriate pH for use in in vitro peptic digestions is difficult since the pH in the in vivo situation is quite variable. However, it is generally accepted that ingestion of food stimulates gastric acid secretion and that gastric acidity is one factor involved in the regulation of gastric acid secretion. Malagelada et al. (16) showed that ingestion of a meal by human subjects increased gastric pH from about 2 to about 5. The peak pH of a 5 was reached rapidly. It then gradually fell with time and stabilized at pH 1.5 to 2 by the end of the second hour. Walsh et al. (17) found that the rate of gastric acid secretion in normal human subjects in response to a meal is suppressed at a gastric pH of 2.5 compared to a gastric pH of 5.5. This suggests that the stomach "titrates" its contents to an acid pH and that stomach pHs following different meals should be similar. It seems reasonable, therefore, to assume that adjustment of the pH to 2 prior to in vitro pepsin digestion would approximate the in vivo situation.

Ferrous and ferric ions are present in the hydrated form in

acidic aqueous solutions (18). As the pH of a solution of these aquated ions is increased, deprotonation of the complexed water molecules occurs and hydroxo- and/or oxo-aquo species are formed (19). This process is called hydrolysis and may be represented as (19)

$$x[Fe(H_2O)_6]^{3+} + y\ H_2O \rightarrow [Fe_x(OH)_y(H_2O)_n]^{(3x-y)+} + y\ H_3O^+$$

where n is the degree of hydration of the hydrolysis product. As the above equation suggests, polynucleated species may be produced in the reaction. Polymers with a molecular weight of 150,000 have been observed (19). Chelating agents such as citrate may prevent polymerization if added in sufficient excess (19). Many of the chelates are, however, quite unstable and addition of concentrated base can cause precipitation even when chelating ligands are present. Upward pH adjustment with $NaHCO_3$ rather than NaOH appears to be less likely to cause precipitation (20).

As the iron is released from food in the acidic environment of the stomach, ligands released in the digestion process combine with the iron to form chelates. These chelates should inhibit polymerization and precipitation of iron as the stomach contents are neutralized in the duodenum provided that localized regions of high pH caused by too rapid addition of concentrated base are avoided. This suggests that pH adjustment in an in vitro simulation is a critical step.

When the products of gastric digestion reach the duodenum, bicarbonate secreted by the pancreas begins to neutralize the stomach acid. The concentration of bicarbonate in pancreatic juice ranges from about 70 to about 150 meq/ℓ (21). In a study involving human subjects, Murthy et al. (22) found the pH of duodenal aspirates to range from 4.7 to 7.2 following administration of a Lundh Test meal.

Selection of appropriate concentrations for digestive enzymes is a difficult undertaking. A large range of concentrations used in in vitro studies have been reported. Akeson and Stahmann (23) used 15 mg pepsin and 40 mg pancreatin per gram of protein. Narasinga Rao and Prabhavathi (11) used pepsin concentrations ranging from 12 to 60 mg per g of food. They reported no difference in iron release when this range of pepsin concentrations was used. Lease (24) used 20 mg of pepsin per gram of food. Hazell et al. (12) used 10 mg pepsin and 10 mg pancreatin per gram of protein. While different concentrations of enzymes will produce different rates of digestion, the actual enzyme concentrations are not critical provided they are precisely duplicated when comparisons between foods or meals are being made.

Appropriate digestion times for an in vitro system likewise cannot be determined with precision. Rates of passage of digesta are determined by several interacting factors including the osmolarity of the meal, the relative amounts of liquid and solid in the meal, the size of the meal and the carbohydrate, protein, and fat content of the meal (25). However, choice of an appropriate pepsin digestion time may be based on estimates of stomach emptying times and rates of digestion. Grimes and Goddard (26) showed that, following a bread and water meal, about 70% of the solid phase (bread) and from 1 to 30% of the liquid phase (water) remained in the stomach one hour after the meal was consumed by human subjects. Malagelada et al. (16) showed with human subjects that gastric volume rose quickly to the volume of the meal and remained at that volume for about one hour. The gastric volume then fell gradually until it reached basal levels about 3 hours from the time the meal was consumed. Narasingao Rao and Prabhavathi showed in an in vitro system that iron released from food was the same when pepsin incubation times were varied from 50 to 180 minutes. Selecton of an in vitro pancreatin digestion time is even more difficult since digesta is constantly entering and leaving the duodenum and jejunum. It is reasonable to select a digestion time that produces significant digestion. Care must be taken to use identical digestion times when comparisons are being made between foods or meals.

Once the conditions for an in vitro method for estimation of iron availability have been established, selection of an appropriate response parameter must be made. Total soluble or "ionizable" iron present in the filtrate or supernate obtained from an in vitro digestion has been the most frequently used response parameter (10-13).

The foregoing discussion provides a basis for selection of a reliable indicator of iron availability. Figure 1 summarizes in schematic form the changes that occur as food moves through the digestive tract. The assumption is made that absorbable iron is present in the duodenum as a low molecular weight soluble chelate. It is further assumed that the other forms of iron that may be present do not contribute significantly to absorbable iron. These assumptions seem justified for the following reasons:

1. Iron may be absorbed as the intact chelate or the chelate may transfer its iron to an acceptor on the mucosal cell surface. Absorption and exchange would be much more rapid with soluble forms of iron since insoluble forms would have limited contact with the mucosal cell surface.
2. Iron bound to large molecular weight ligands may be available but absorption would be limited to an iron transfer mechanism since large molecules are generally not absorbed intact. Large molecular weight soluble chelates of available iron would most likely involve proteins as the ligand and digestion would quickly transform them into low molecular weight chelates.
3. Polymerized iron, even when soluble, is probably not readily available. Bates et al. (20), in studies designed to measure iron exchange rates between chelates and transferrin, showed that polymerized iron was transferred to transferrin

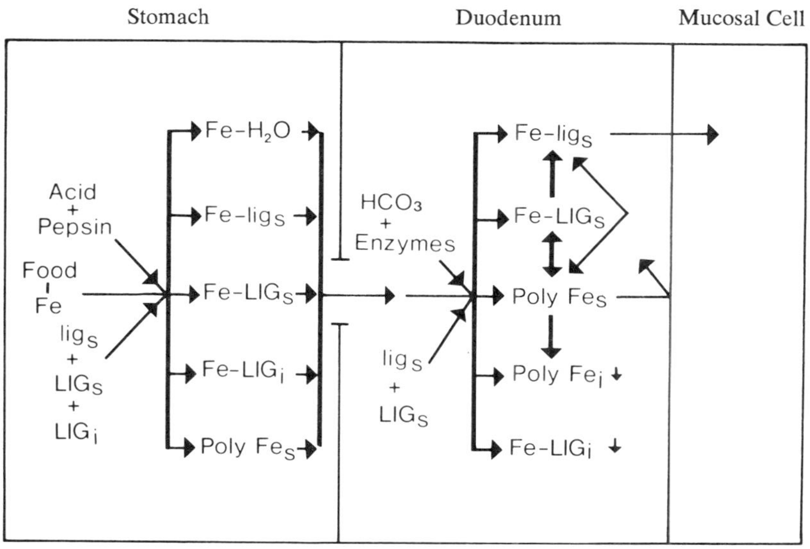

Figure 1. Proposed model for changes that occur in nonheme iron as food moves through GI tract. Abbreviations: lig_s, low molecular weight soluble ligand; LIG_s, large molecular weight soluble ligand; LIG_i, large molecular weight insoluble ligand; Poly Fe_s, soluble polynuclear (polymerized) iron; Poly Fe_i, insoluble polynuclear (polymerized) iron.

at a very slow rate while iron in the low molecular weight nitrilotriacetate chelate was almost instantaneously transferred to the transferrin. Polymerized iron may be depolymerized by ligands and/or reducing agents (27) and thereby enter the low molecular weight iron chelate pool.

Consideration of the factors discussed above provides a reasonably good rationale for the design of an in vitro method to estimate food iron availability. Briefly, it seems apparent that an in vitro method should:

1. Simulate in vivo digestion conditions.
2. Permit pH control.
3. Provide for gradual pH adjustment with a mild base.
4. Distinguish between low and high molecular weight soluble iron.
5. Accommodate food mixtures (meals).

Description of the Method

Details of the method have been described elsewhere (28,29). A flow diagram of the method is shown in Figure 2. Briefly, the method involves the following steps:

1. Water is added to mixtures of foods (meals) so that the water content of different meals is approximately the same.
2. The meals are blended in a food blender to a creamy consistency.
3. The pH of the blended meals is adjusted to 2 with 6 N HCl and the samples are spiked with ^{59}Fe.
4. Pepsin is added and the meals are incubated in a shaking water bath at 37°C for 2 hours.
5. Aliquots of the pepsin digest are analyzed for a) titratable acidity (the number of equivalents of KOH required to titrate a 20 g aliquot containing 5 ml of the pancreatin-bile mixture to pH 7.5), b) nonheme iron concentration, and c) ^{59}Fe activity.
6. A dialysis bag containing an amount of $NaHCO_3$ in 25 ml of water equivalent to the previously determined titratable acidity is added to a 20 g aliquot of the pepsin digest. The sample is incubated for 30 minutes at 37°C in a shaking water bath. During this time, the pH increases to about 5.
7. Five ml of a pancreatin-bile acid mixture is added to each digestion vessel (it is added to the contents outside the dialysis bag). Incubation is continued for 2 hours.
8. The dialysis bag is removed, rinsed in distilled water, and emptied of its contents (the dialysate).
9. The dialysate is weighed and analyzed for ^{59}Fe activity and bathophenanthroline reactive iron.
10. Results are expressed as percent of total nonheme and radioiron in the original aliquot that is present in the dialysis bag at the end of the digestion.

In order to evaluate the method, meals were prepared that

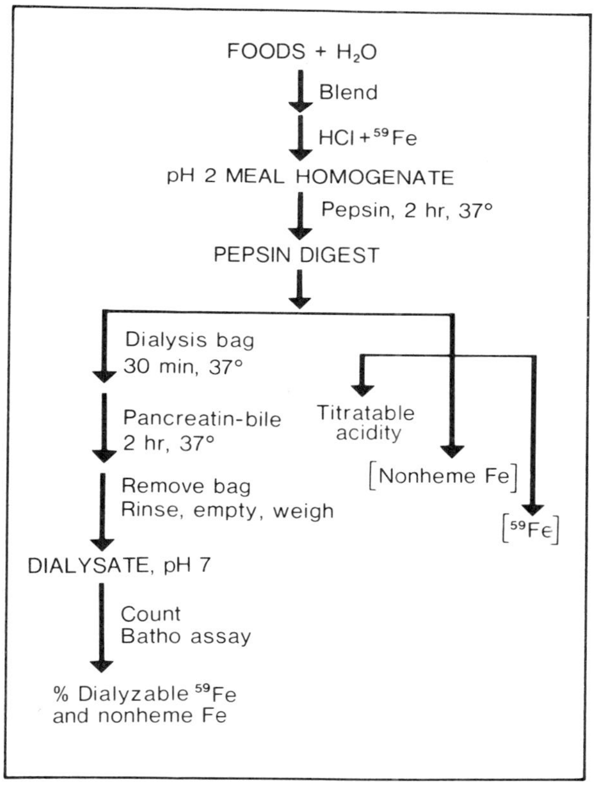

Figure 2. Schematic of the in vitro method. See text for details.

would permit food substitutions that might alter levels of dialyzable iron. One meal was of our own formulation (the standard meal) and two were replicates of meals used by Cook and Monsen (7,30). The composition of these meals is shown in Table I.

Table I: Composition of Test Meals Used in Iron Availability Trials*

Standard	STD, Cook & Monsen	SS, Cook & Monsen
Beef; lean ground	Beef; ground	Albumin; egg
Bread; white, enriched	Potatoes; dry	Dextrose
	Cornmeal	Corn oil
Beans; snap, frozen	Bread; white, enriched	$CaHPO_4$
Milk; fluid, whole	Margarine	K_2HPO_4
Water	Peaches	Fe solution
	Ice milk	Water
	Water	

*The STD and SS meals were originally formulated by Cook and Monsen (7,30).

Results and Evaluation

The 2 hour pepsin incubation time was based on work reported by Narasinga Rao (11) and on literature reports on gastric emptying time (16,26). The slightly longer pancreatin incubation time of 2 1/2 hours was chosen for two reasons. First, it was necessary to delay addition of the pancreatin-bile mixture for 30 minutes after the dialysis bag was added and the incubation begun. The delay allowed the pH to rise to about 5 and thereby prevented inactivation of the pancreatic enzymes which does occur at lower pHs (22). Secondly, this time period produced sufficient dialysate iron concentrations for accurate bathophenanthroline measurements. Figure 3 shows a time course for dialyzable iron changes during the second incubation. Dialyzable iron rises rapidly to equilibrium levels when the semisynthetic meal is used. This suggests that pancreatin digestion has little effect on available iron in a meal composed of purified ingredients. For the standard meal, on the other hand, dialyzable iron increases steadily over the entire incubation period. This suggests that digestion by pancreatic enzymes does play a role in food iron availability.

Data from Malagelada et al. (16) provided the basis for choosing a pH of 2 for the pepsin digestion. A final dialysate pH of 7 was chosen for the pancreatin digestion on the basis of the data of Murthy et al. (22). Attempts were made to adjust the

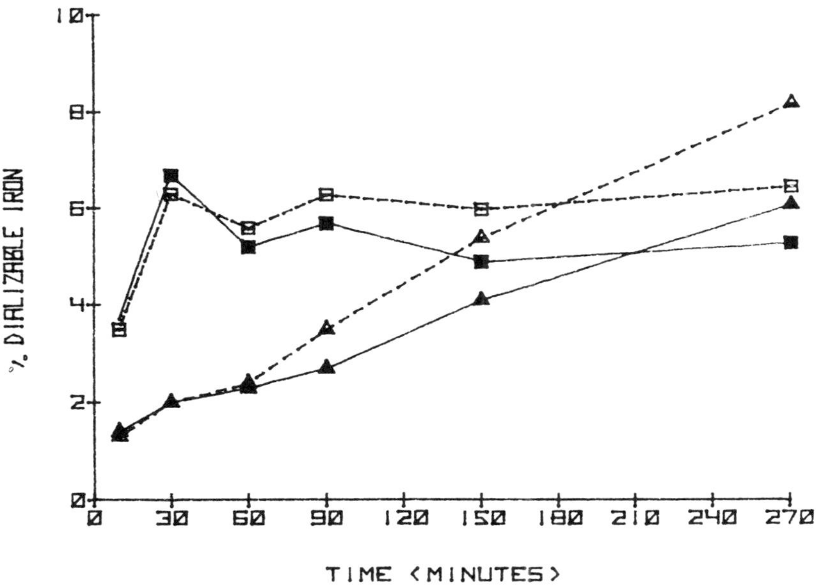

Figure 3. Time course for changes in dialyzable iron during the second digestion step. See text for a description of meals and digestion conditions. Key: ▲, standard, colorimetric; △, standard, radioactive; ■, SS, colorimetric; □, SS, radioactive.

pH of the pepsin digest by dropwise addition of dilute $NaHCO_3$ or NaOH but this approach produced variable and poorly reproducible values for dialyzable iron. Adjustment of pH by dialysis produced the least variable and most reproducible dialyzable iron values. In addition, this method of pH adjustment permits dialysis of iron to occur during the neutralization process, a situation which more closely resembles the in vivo process. Even with this method of pH adjustment, however, the final dialysate pHs did vary. In order to determine the effect of variation in final pH on dialyzable iron, an experiment was run using different amounts of bicarbonate in the dialysis bags. The amounts used were based on titratable acidity measurements made with different end points. Aliquots were titrated to final pHs ranging from 6.5 to 8.5. Addition of $NaHCO_3$ based on these titrations produced final dialysate pHs ranging from about 6 to about 7.5. Figure 4 shows that in the range of pH variability observed when different meals are run in the in vitro procedure (final pHs in the acidity titration of 7.0 to 8.0), the effect of pH on dialyzable iron is small. It is interesting to note that the direction of pH effects are different for the semisynthetic and standard meals. The decrease observed with increasing pH in the semisynthetic meal would be expected if digestion were not a factor since higher pHs would cause increased formation of polymerized iron. The increase observed in the standard meal can be explained by an increase in pancreatic enzyme activity at higher pHs.

Table II shows effects on dialyzable iron caused by various substitution into the standard meal. These data have been reported elsewhere (Miller et al. 28, Schricker et al. 29).

Table II: Percent Dialyzable Iron[*,†], Effects of Selected Foods

Substitution	Colorimetric	Radioactive
None, Standard meal	4.08 ± 0.31^{a}	3.80 ± 0.31^{a}
Ham for beef	5.05 ± 0.80^{a}	5.14 ± 0.23^{a}
Whole wheat for white bread	2.06 ± 0.42^{b}	1.49 ± 0.10^{b}
Spinach for green beans	5.73 ± 0.33^{a}	5.04 ± 0.19^{a}
Water for milk	4.59 ± 0.32^{ac}	4.16 ± 0.14^{a}
Tea for milk	2.80 ± 0.31^{b}	1.52 ± 0.21^{b}
Cola for milk	6.14 ± 0.61^{c}	7.82 ± 0.34^{c}
Orange juice for milk	24.96 ± 0.83^{d}	25.83 ± 0.86^{d}

* Values represent means ± S.E. for three observations.

† In each column, means followed by different superscripts are significantly different (P<0.01).

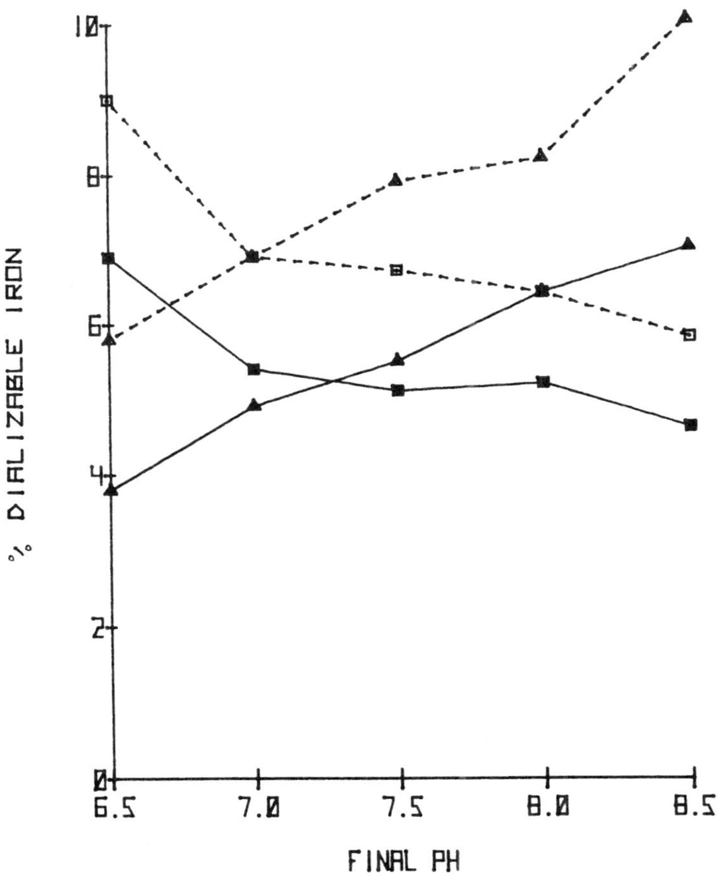

Figure 4. Effect of pH on dialyzable iron. Values on x axis are endpoints for the titratable acidity measurement. Final pH of dialysate after incubation about 0.5 below the pH shown. Key: ▲, standard, colorimetric; △, standard, radioactive; ■, SS, colorimetric; □, SS, radioactive.

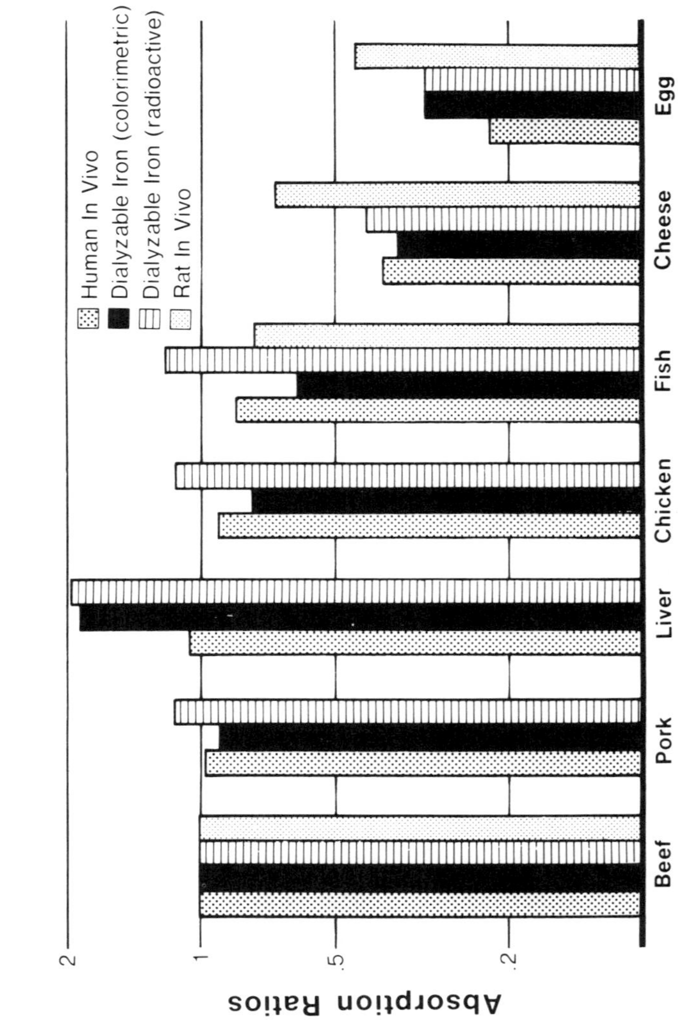

Figure 5. Comparison of estimated absorption ratios for standard meals using different methodology. All meals are compared to the beef meal. Ratios for human in vivo trials are derived from data from Cook and Monsen (7). Ratios are plotted on a logarithmic scale.

To further evaluate the method, a series of meals were formulated and prepared to duplicate those of Cook and Monsen (7) (see Table I). These meals were chosen because they were used by Cook and Monsen in a study involving human subjects and, therefore, provided a means for comparison of in vitro and human in vivo methods. A rat in vivo method was also used in this study. The meals were homogenized, spiked with ^{59}Fe, and administered to rats via stomach tube. Iron retention was measured using whole body counting. Figure 5 compares results obtained using these three methods.

Comparison of results from the in vitro and human in vivo methods shows good agreement between the two methods.

On the basis of the description and results presented above, it is reasonable to characterize the in vitro method described here as:

1. Rapid and inexpensive
2. Reproducible
3. A good predictor of relative iron bioavailability
4. Potentially useful for:
   a. Food iron availability screening
   b. Identifying factors and mechanisms which may influence iron availability

Literature Cited

1. Monsen, E.R.; Hallberg, L.; Layrisse, M.; Hegsted, D.M.; Cook, J.D.; Mertz, W.; Finch, C.A. Am. J. Clin. Nutr. 1978, 31, 134-141.
2. Fritz, J.C.; Pla, G.W.; Harrison, B.M.; Clark, G.A.; Smith, E.A. J. Assoc. Off. Anal. Chem. 1978, 61, 709-714.
3. Miller, J. J. Agric. Food Chem. 1977, 25, 154-158.
4. Rotruck, J.T.; Luhrsen, K.R. J. Agric. Food Chem. 1979, 27, 27-33.
5. Welch, R.M.; Van Campen, R. J. Nutr. 1975, 105, 253-256.
6. Hallberg, L. Proc. Nutr. Soc. 1974, 33, 285-291.
7. Cook, J.D.; Monsen, E.R. Am. J. Clin. Nutr. 1976, 29, 859-867.
8. Shackleton,L.; McCance, R.A. Biochem. J. 1936, 30, 583-591.
9. Lee, K. Clydesdale, F.M J. Food Sci. 1979, 44, 549-554.
10. Jacobs, A.; Greenman, D.A. Brit. Med. J. 1969, 1, 673-676.
11. Narasinga Rao, B.S.; Prabhavathi, T. Am. J. Clin. Nutr. 1978, 31, 169-175.
12. Hazell, T.; Ledward, D.A.; Neal, R.J. Br. J. Nutr. 1978, 39, 631-638.
13. Lock, S.; Bender, A.E. Br. J. Nutr. 1980, 43, 413-420.
14. Forth, W.; Rummel, W. Physiol. Rev. 1973, 53, 724-792.
15. Bezwoda, W.; Charlton, R.; Bothwell, T.; Torrance, J.; Mayet, F. J. Lab. Clin. Med. 1978, 92, 108-116.
16. Malagelada, J.; Go, Longstreth, G.F.; Deering, T.B.; Summerskill, W.H.J.; Go, V.L.W. Gastroenterology. 1977, 73, 989-994.

17. Walsh, J.H.; Richardson, C.T.; Fordtran, J.S. J. Clin. Invest. 1975, 55, 462-468.
18. Spiro, T.G.; Saltman, P. In: Jacobs, A.; Worwood, M., Eds.; "Iron in Biochemistry and Medicine"; Academic Press: New York, NY, 1974; pp 1-28.
19. Sylva, R.N. Rev. Pure and Appl. Chem. 1972, 22, 115-132.
20. Bates, G.W.; Billups, C.; Saltman, P. J. Biol. Chem. 1967, 242, 2810-2815.
21. Ganong, W.F. "Review of Medical Physiology", 6th ed.; Lang Medical Publications: Los Altos, CA, 1973; p 370.
22. Murthy, S.N.S.; Kostman, J.; Dinoso, V.P. Dig. Dis. Sci., 1980, 25, 289-294.
23. Akeson, W.R.; Stahmann, M.A. J. Nutr. 1964, 83, 257-261.
24. Lease, J.G. J. Nutr. 1967, 93, 523-532.
25. Fein, H.D. In: Goodhart, R.S.; Shils, M.E., Eds.; "Modern Nutrition in Health and Disease", 6th ed.; Lea and Febiger: Philadelphia, PA, 1980; p 894.
26. Grimes, D.S.; Goddard, J. Gut. 1977, 18, 725-729.
27. Saltman, P.; Hegenaur, J.; Christopher, J. Ann. Clin. Lab. Sci. 1976, 6, 167-176.
28. Miller, D.D.; Schricker, B.R.; Rasmussen, R.R.; Van Campen, D. Am. J. Clin. Nutr. 1981, 34, 2248-2256.
29. Schricker, B.R.; Miller, D.D.; Rasmussen, R.R.; Van Campen, D. Am. J. Clin. Nutr. 1981, 34, 2257-2263.
30. Cook, J.D.; Monsen, E.R. Am. J. Clin. Nutr. 1975, 28, 1289-1295.

RECEIVED June 2, 1982.

3

Iron Chemistry and Bioavailability in Food Processing

KENNETH LEE

University of Wisconsin-Madison, Department of Food Science, Madison, WI 53706

The effect of food processing on the bioavailability and chemistry of iron was reviewed with emphasis on research employing an iron profile analysis. Iron profiling, a measurement of iron valence, solubility, and complexation, identified chemical changes which took place in drying, baking and retort processes. Agreement between iron profile and animal bioavailability data was observed. A distinction between wet-heat versus dry-heat processing was drawn which may account for some of the differences found in research on the effect of heat processing on iron bioavailability. The effect of added chemicals, including ascorbic acid and sodium ferric EDTA, were also considered. The studies reviewed collectively suggest that iron bioavailability depended upon the iron source, the food matrix and the type of food process. Measuring chemical changes in endogenous or added iron in foods after processing will help evaluate changes in iron bioavailability due to food processing.

Both food processing and iron chemistry are important factors affecting iron bioavailability. The chemistry of iron, particularly its valence, solubility and type of chelation, may influence the absorption of iron. Several dietary studies have shown changes in iron bioavailability as a result of various forms of food processing. These process-induced changes in bioavailability may correspond to a change in the chemistry of iron. There are also some data which show that iron chemistry changes after some forms of food processing. This supports the idea that a food or food process can be "chemically optimized" to yield the best possible bioavailability of iron.

Processes such as baking, canning, curing or cooking all have been examined for a nutritional effect on iron. In most cases, the bioavailability of iron was changed, increasing in some cases and decreasing in others. What caused these changes in bioavailability? Were there absorption enhancers or

0097-6156/82/0203-0027$08.00/0

inhibitors produced or removed by the process? Was the chemistry of the iron itself altered in some way? Answers may reveal how food controls the bioavailability of iron. Correlation of chemical indices with bioavailability may enable rapid optimization of a food for the most desirable iron availability.

This chapter mentions some iron chemistry important to its bioavailability and the changes which may be induced by food processing. The reader may refer to the chapter by Spiro and Saltman (1) for a discussion of inorganic iron chemistry. This author has critically reviewed the iron sources used for food enrichment earlier (2). A good review of the chemistry of iron in myoglobin has been published by Livingston and Brown (3). Forth and Rummel (4) have made available an extensive review on iron absorption and factors which affect iron absorption. Waddell reviewed the iron enrichment program in the United States and the bioavailability of iron sources (5).

Food Processing

It may be useful to consider what is meant by "food processing", for the term is used in many ways. Nearly all rat studies utilize one common form of food processing, i.e. freeze drying for feed preparation. Even this rather mild form of processing may affect iron, as atmospheric oxidation of freeze dried beef decreased iron bioavailability from beef (6). Many studies on the effect of "processing" actually employed only heat processing. Heating is a major form, but not the only form of processing which may affect the nutritional value of iron.

Addition or removal of energy, microorganisms, or chemicals, and food rearrangements are seven major ways in which food is processed (Table I). Each of these processes can affect the bioavailability of iron. Most iron bioavailability research has focused upon the first and the fifth categories, addition of energy and addition of chemicals. The remaining forms of food processing leave an interesting area which remains to be evaluated for chemical and nutritional effects on mineral nutrition.

Iron Sources

It is sometimes the practice in the food industry to add the most bioavailable iron salt at the last practical processing step, with the hope of maintaining iron bioavailability with no sacrifice in product quality. For example, ferrous sulfate is sometimes used at the bakery level for enriching flour during dough formulation. It is not added to the flour at the mill because ferrous sulfate is a prooxidant and can cause rancidity and off flavors (7). The less reactive and more flour compatible iron phosphates are sometimes avoided, based upon research which show the iron phosphates are not bioavailable. The preference for one iron source over another stems from their relative ranking in terms of biological values, as shown in Table II.

Table I. Classification of major forms of food processing.

	Type of Process	Some Examples
1.	Add Energy	Cooking, irridation, pasteurization, heating
2.	Remove Energy	Refrigeration, freezing
3.	Add Microorganisms	Fermentation, curing, aging
4.	Remove Microorganisms	Cleaning, sorting
5.	Add Chemicals	Dilution, fortification, additives, pickling
6.	Remove Chemicals	Extraction, dehydration, distillation, detoxification
7.	Rearrangements	Homogenization, emulsification, gelation, blending, enzymatic conversions, packaging

Table II. Iron sources currently used in food enrichment and their relative biological values (RBV) based upon direct feeding.

Iron Source	RBV*	Compatability with foods
Ferrous sulfate	100	very poor
Ferrous gluconate	97	
Ferrous fumarate	95	
Electrolytic-type elemental iron	45-76	
Carbonyl process elemental iron	64-69	
Hydrogen reduced elemental iron	18-54	
Ferric sodium pyrophosphate	14	
Ferric ortho phosphate	3-46	very good

*As reported by Fritz et al. (8).

An extensive series of studies performed at the FDA Division of Nutrition established a wide range of bioavailabilities for the iron sources used in food enrichment (8-12). However, the rank in Table II was based on direct feeding of the iron source to test animals. The impact of food processing or of the food matrix on iron bioavailability is not apparent in these rankings. Large differences in bioavailability between iron sources will become smaller or change completely as a result of some types of processing, while other processes have little effect.

Effect of Heat Processing on Iron Bioavailability

Addition of energy in the form of heat has been shown in a number of studies to dramatically influence iron bioavailability. Heating did not consistently enhance iron absorption, in some cases heating was inhibitory when compared to an unheated control. Whether or not the available iron increased, decreased, or stayed the same appeared to depend on two major factors: 1) the food or chemical matrix in which the iron resided, and 2) the identity of the iron source added. Some studies which illustrated these points are summarized in Table III.

Effect of Heat Processing on Bioavailability of Added Iron. Several studies in Table III measured directly the effect of heat processing on added iron. These studies compared processed foods to a control group of identical unprocessed food. Studies in Table III utilizing unprocessed controls include 15, 19, and 23. Other studies did not employ an unprocessed control, but used a reference dose to enable comparisons from study to study. Reference doses of ferrous sulfate (most animal assays) or ferrous ascorbate (most human tests) were frequently used. Preparation of ferrous ascorbate, usually a 2:1 molar ascorbic acid:iron solution, has been detailed by Layrisse et al. (25). These controls enabled measurement of variation in iron absorption from subject to subject, important in view of greater absorption of an iron deficient versus an iron replete subject. When a reference dose was fed as a radiolabeled salt (55Fe), and on alternate times the test diet was fed with a different radiolabel (59Fe), errors due to variation in subject absorption were eliminated, as each subject served as its own control. The different availabilities of various iron sources from baked enriched rolls were established in this manner (17).

A few trends are evident from the heat-processing data in Table III. Processing increased bioavailability of added iron when the process involved heating a predominantly aqueous food (i.e., wet-heat processing), as well as when ascorbic acid was added before heating. A greater bioavailability resulted after the processing of canned liquid milk-based infant formula (13),

Table III. Some studies which examined the effect of heat processing on the bioavailability of iron added to foods.

Processed Food	Type of Iron Added to Food	Control	Bioavailability of added iron vs. Control	Test Type & (species)*	Reference
Canned liquid soy-isolate infant formula	Ferric pyrophosphate Ferric sodium pyrophosphate	$FeSO_4$	Greater	Repletion (rat)	13
Canned liquid milk-based infant formula	Ferric pyrophosphate Ferric sodium pyrophosphate $FeSO_4$	$FeSO_4$	Greater	Repletion (rat)	14
Canned experimental milk-based liquid	Elemental iron Carbonyl iron	Unprocessed	Greater	Repletion (rat)	15
Canned experimental milk-based liquid	Ferric ortho phosphate	Unprocessed	No change	Repletion (rat)	15
Processed bran breakfast cereal	Elemental iron Carbonyl iron H_2 reduced iron	Semipurified diets	No change	Repletion (rat)	16
Baked yeast-leavened rolls	Sodium ferric pyrophosphate Ferric ortho phosphate $FeSO_4$	Ferrous ascorbate	Less	Extrinsic (human)	17
Baked yeast-leavened rolls	$FeSO_4$ H_2 reduced iron	Ferrous ascorbate	No change	Extrinsic (human)	17
Baked yeast-leavened bread	Ferric ammonium citrate Ferrum redactum	Ferrous ascorbate	Less	Extrincic (human)	18
Cooked corn-meal cereal fortified with ascorbic acid	$FePO_4 \cdot H_2O$ added before cooking	$FePO_4 \cdot H_2O$ added after cooking	Greater	Intrinsic-extrinsic (women)	19

Continued on next page.

Table III, continued

Processed Food	Type of Iron Added to Food	Control	Bioavailability of added iron vs. Control	Test Type & (species)*	Reference
Cooked fortified apple jam on white bread	$FePO_4 \cdot H_2O$ cooked with ascorbic acid	$FePO_4$ H_2O cooked without ascorbic acid	Greater	Intrinsic-extrinsic (women)	19
Baked enriched soda crackers	Reduced iron enriched crackers	$FeSO_4$ enriched crackers	Less	Repletion (rat)	20
Baked commercial variety breads	$FeSO_4$ enriched reduced iron enriched or unenriched breads	$FeSO_4$	Less	Repletion (rat)	21
Processed (heat, enzyme, air-dry) mixed grain infant cereal	Reduced iron Ferric ortho phosphate, or Sodium ferric pyrophosphate enriched cereals	$FeSO_4$ enriched cereal	Less	Extrinsic (rat)	22
Retorted, chopped air-dried lab diet	$Fe_4(P_2O_7)_3 \cdot 9H_2O$ $Fe_4Na_8O_{35}P_{10}$	Unprocessed diet	No change	Repletion (chick)	23
Retorted, chopped, air-dried lab diet	$FeSO_4$	Unprocessed diet	Greater	Repletion (chick)	23
Cooked corn cereal	Ferric ammonium citrate and ascorbic acid added before cooking	No iron or ascorbic acid added	Greater	Intrinsic-extrinsic (human)	24
Baked whole-wheat bread	Ferric ammonium citrate and ascorbic acid added before cooking	No iron or ascorbic acid added	Less	Intrinsic-extrinsic (human)	24

*Test types are as follows: Repletion; hemoglobin or hematocrit repletion by the test sample of iron was measured in animals first made anemic. Extrinsic; a soluble radioiron salt label was used to mark the nonheme iron pool. Extrinsic-intrinsic; both an added iron salt and the endogenous food iron were radiolabeled with 55Fe and 59Fe.

canned liquid soy-based infant formula (14), canned milk-based beverage (15), boiled corn cereal (19), retorted milk-corn slurry diets (23), and the cooking of corn cereal with added ascorbic acid (24). The above studies employed various iron sources which all increased in availability except in two studies; ferric ortho phosphate, an extremely insoluble iron source, remained unchanged (15), and ferrous sulfate was unaffected (23).

Dry-heat processing had little effect on the bioavailability of added iron. No change in bioavailability was observed after the baking of yeast leavened rolls (17), yeast leavened bread (18), enriched soda crackers (20), commercial variety breads (21), whole-wheat breads (24), or processed infant cereals (22). Differences in bioavailability due to the process of baking *per se* cannot be discerned, as these studies used a baked, ferrous sulfate enriched control. A ferrous sulfate enriched control highlighted differences between iron sources rather than effects of baking. As seen in Table III, the bioavailability of iron in baked goods depended upon the iron source used for enrichment. In general, ferrous sulfate was superior in availability both before and after baking. In a human study, the absorption of ferrous sulfate baked into bread or rolls ranged from 3.6% to 9.1%, roughly one-fourth the level observed when ferrous sulfate was given as a solution of inorganic iron (17). This level of absorption is similar to the availability of endogenous iron reported by Layrisse et al. (25) for most vegetable foods, but less than the iron from meats or soy, shown in Table IV.

Effect of Heat Processing on the Bioavailability of Iron Naturally Present. Bioavailability of iron naturally present in foods depended upon the nature of the process and the accompanying food matrix (Table IV). Iron in cooked corn cereal, a wet-heat process, increased in bioavailability when cooked along with ascorbic acid (24). However, iron in baked soy biscuits or baked bread, both dry-heat processes, did not change in bioavailability when cooked along with ascorbic acid (24). Data from South Africa, where the Bantu people suffer from siderosis, a chronic iron overload, show that the iron in beer commonly consumed was over 12 times more bioavailable than iron from a gruel of the beer ingredients (26). Derman et al. postulated that lactic acid, produced in brewing, acted as a chelator which enhanced iron absorption (26). Rotruck and Luhrsen found that bioavailability was greatest with ferrous sulfate, followed by soy protein isolate, processed soy protein, then cooked beef, also in Table IV (27). These authors point out that soy protein iron bioavailability was equal or nearly equal to ferrous sulfate. This is contrary to recent human data which has shown soy to be inhibitory (28). Measurement of the chemical differences in the soy preparations may be helpful in accounting for

Table IV. Some studies which examined the effect of heat processing on the bioavailability of iron naturally present in foods.

Processed Food	% Absorption From Control¶	% Absorption from Processed Food	Bioavailability After Processing vs. Control	Test Type (species)*	Reference
Baked yeast-leavened dinner rolls	Ferrous ascorbate	4.9% wheat 55Fe 6.1% $FeSO_4$ tag	Less	Intrinsic-extrinsic (human)	17
Grilled corn pancakes (arepas)	40.3% Ferrous ascorbate	5.9% corn 55Fe	Less	Intrinsic (human)	25
Boiled black beans	21.4% Ferrous ascorbate	3.2% bean 55Fe	Less	Intrinsic (human)	25
Boiled then baked soybean flour	34.3% Ferrous ascorbate	17.9% soy 55Fe	Less	Intrinsic (human)	25
Fried sweet fish	44.8% Ferrous ascorbate	18.3% fish 55Fe	Less	Intrinsic (human)	25
Cooked veal	19.7% Ferrous ascorbate	20.3% veal 55Fe	No change	Intrinsic (human)	25
Cooked corn cereal	Cooked without ascorbic acid: 3.8% corn 55Fe, 6.8% 59Fe tag	Cooked with 50 mg added ascorbic acid 14.9% corn 55Fe, 23.7 59Fe tag	Greater	Intrinsic extrinsic (human)	24
Baked soy biscuits	Baked without ascorbic acid: 19.8% soy 55Fe, 21.1% 59Fe tag	Baked with 100 mg ascorbic acid: 14.6% soy 55Fe 15.5% 59Fe tag	No change	Intrinsic extrinsic (human)	24

Processed Food	% Absorption From Control¶	% Absorption from Processed Food	Bioavailability After Processing vs. Control	Test Type (species)*	Reference
Baked whole-wheat bread	Baked with ascorbic acid: 7.9% whole wheat 55Fe, 9.0% 59Fe tag	Baked with 50 mg ascorbic acid: 6.6% wheat iron 10.0% extrinsic tag	No change	Intrinsic-extrinsic (human)	24
Brewed corn & sorgum beer (malted, fermented, boiled, fermented, filtered)	0.6% absorption from gruel of pre-brew ingredients	7.7% absorption from brewed beer	Greater	Extrinsic (human)	26
Baked chuck roast (beef)	$FeSO_4$	Beef iron	Less	Repletion (rat)	27
Processed soybean protein isolate	$FeSO_4$	Soy iron	No change	Repletion (rat)	27
Soybean protein isolate	$FeSO_4$	Soy iron	No change	Repletion (rat)	27
Nitrite cured beef (bologna)	Nitrite free bologna	Nitrite cured beef	Less	Repletion (rat)	6

*Test types are as follows: Repletion; hemoglobin or hematocrit repletion by the test sample of iron was measured in animals first made anemic. Extrinsic; a soluble radioiron salt label was used to mark the nonheme iron pool. Intrinsic; foods were grown with a radioiron maker to label the iron *in situ*. Extrinsic-Intrinsic; both an added iron salt and the endogenous food iron were radiolabeled with 55Fe and 59Fe.

¶Percentages refer to the mean percent of the total dose absorbed by subjects.

the contrasting results. The addition of nitrite to beef was shown to inhibit iron absorption in rats, correlating well with water-extractable iron (6). However, as nitrite levels increased above 50 mg/kg meat the iron utilization improved, indicating a second mechanism which remains to be elucidated.

Effect of Organic Acids and Carbohydrates on Iron Bioavailability

Several chemicals added to foods have been investigated for their effect on iron absorption, as listed in Table V. Organic acids and sugars have been shown capable of affecting iron bioavailability. It is of interest to note that these acids and sugars are also capable of forming soluble chelates with iron.

Organic Acids. Ascorbic acid has been most extensively studied and its absorption promoting property is well documented (Table V). Ascorbic acid has been shown to increase iron uptake in proportion to its concentration in the diet (29). Tea inhibited iron absorption from a corn-cereal diet, but supplementation with ascorbic acid overcame the inhibition (30). Ascorbic acid also increased the absorption of iron from fairly insoluble forms of iron such as rust and ferric hydroxide (30). Brise and Hallberg presented evidence that the absorption promoting effect of ascorbic acid was mainly due to reducing action within the lumen, preventing or delaying formation of less soluble ferric compounds (31). Conrad and Schade (32) found that ascorbic acid formed a soluble chelate with ferric chloride at an acid pH, but not at an alkaline pH. However, the acid iron chelate was stable and remained in a soluble form when the pH was raised.

Several other organic acids which modify iron absorption are also listed in Table V. EDTA has received much attention for it forms a highly stable iron chelate, and one would expect it to inhibit iron absorption. When sodium ferric EDTA (NaFeEDTA) was fed directly as a liquid, inhibition of iron absorption was observed both in rats (4) and in man (40, 48). Inhibition increased with increasing chelate concentration. This effect was also observed when NaFeEDTA was added to a diet, but only when the molar ratio of disodium EDTA to iron was 2:1 or greater (33). The inhibition was observed when NaFeEDTA was added to a standard meal described as "a typical American dinner," or when it was added to a semisynthetic meal (a diet designed to yield low iron bioavailability) (33).

Other studies listed in Table V support the belief that NaFeEDTA may be a good iron enrichment source. Sugar was investigated as a carrier for iron. NaFeEDTA with sugar was greater in bioavailability to humans than ferrous sulfate (46). NaFeEDTA was functionally superior to ferrous sulfate in that it did not form iron-tannin precipitates when used in tea (46). NaFeEDTA absorption from a standard meal containing radiolabeled

Table V. Studies which examined the effect of addition of organic acids or carbohydrates to food on the bioavailability of iron.

Chemical Added to Food	Level Added¶	Food	Iron Source	Effect of Added Chemical on Iron Bioavailability**	Test Type (species)*	Reference
Organic Acids:						
Ascorbic acid	25-1000 mg	Semisynthetic meal	$FeCl_3$	2-10 times greater absorption	Extrinsic (men)	29
Ascorbic acid	50 mg 100 mg 50 mg 100 mg	Corn-meal cereal Corn-meal cereal Corn-meal & tea Corn-meal & tea	$FeCl_3$ $FeCl_3$ $FeCl_3$ $FeCl_3$	10-fold increase 10-fold increase 2-fold increase 5-fold increase	Extrinsic (women)	30
Ascorbic acid	100 mg	Corn-meal cereal	Fe_2O_3 $Fe(OH)_3$	0.01% to 0.5% increase 1.5% to 6.7% increase	Extrinsic (women)	30
Ascorbic acid	10:1¶ 20:1	Corn-meal cereal Corn-meal cereal	$FeSO_4$ $FeSO_4$	Doubled absorption Tripled absorption	Intrinsic Extrinsic (human)	30
Ascorbic acid	50-500 mg	No food was given	$FeSO_4$	Increased absorption only with 200 mg or more dose	Extrinsic (human)	31
Ascorbic acid	0.01 M	No food was given	$FeCl_2$ $FeCl_3$	11.5% to 19.6% increase 8.9% to 19.1% increase	Extrinsic (rat)	32
Disodium EDTA dihydrate	1:1	Standard meal	$FeCl_3$	No effect	Extrinsic (men)	33
Disodium EDTA dihydrate	2:1 50 mg	Standard meal Semisynthetic meal	$FeCl_3$ $FeCl_3$	1/2 absorption 1.3% to 0.9% decrease	Extrinsic (men)	33
Ferric EDTA	5-50 mg	Standard meal & radiolabeled corn	FeEDTA	Doubled absorption over ferrous sulfate	Intrinsic Extrinsic (human)	34

Continued on next page.

Table V, continued

Chemical Added to Food	Level Added¶	Food	Iron Source	Effect of Added Chemical on Iron Bioavailability**	Test Type (species)*	Reference
Ferric EDTA	3 mg Fe	Standard meal & radiolabeled corn	FeEDTA	9.6% from FeEDTA versus 2.8% from ferrous sulfate	Intrinsic Extrinsic (human)	35
Sodium ferric EDTA	5 mg Fe	Milk-rice-sugar formula mixture	NaFeEDTA	8.6% from NaFeEDTA versus 3.3% from ferric sulfate and 34.5% from hemoglobin	Extrinsic (children)	36
Sodium ferric EDTA	5 mg Fe	Beans, tortillas, bread, & coffee	NaFeEDTA	6.4% from NaFeEDTA versus 2.4% from ferric sulfate	Extrinsic (human)	36
Monoferric phytate	18 ppm	Purified diet	FePhytate	Same as ferrous ammonium sulfate, greater than Fe_2Phytate and Fe_4Phytate	Repletion (rat)	37
Monoferric phytate	2-60 mg Fe	Standard meal	FePhytate	Same bioavailability as $FeCl_3$ tag	Extrinsic (dog)	38
Oxalic acid	0.75%	Low iron diet with 25% freeze-dried spinach	Spinach iron	No effect, possible increase	Intrinsic (rat)	39
Succinic acid	30-500 mg	No food was given	$FeSO_4$	1 to 1.6 fold increase	Extrinsic (human)	40
Fumaric acid	1 millimol	No food was given	$FeSO_4$	No effect	Extrinsic (human)	40
Lactic acid	3 mg per subject	Boiled corn-meal gruel	$FeCl_3$	0.4% from gruel versus 1.2% from gruel + lactate	Extrinsic (human)	26

Chemical Added to Food	Level Added¶	Food	Iron Source	Effect of Added Chemical on Iron Bioavailability**	Test Type (species)*	Reference
Carbohydrates:						
Fructose Fructose	0.4 mMol 0.4 mMol	No food was given No food was given	$FeCl_3$ $FeCl_3$	10.1% to 15.7% increase 18.5% to 19.6% no effect	Extrinsic (rat)	41
Fructose	2.5:1 to 100:1	No food, given as tablets	Ferric fructose	Increased absorption only with 100:1 fructose:iron	Extrinsic (human)	42
Glucose	40% of diet	Purified diet	Ferric sodium pyrophosphate	No effect versus sucrose	Repletion (rat)	43
Glucose	0.04 mMol	No food was given	$FeCl_3$	No effect	Extrinsic (rat)	41
Galactose	0.4 mMol	No food was given	$FeCl_3$	No effect	Extrinsic (rat)	41
Sorbitol	11.7 mg/mg iron	No food was given	$FeSO_4$	1.3 to 2.4 times increase	Extrinsic (human)	44
Lactose	22% of diet	Purified diet	Ferric sodium pyrophosphate	Slight decrease versus sucrose	Repletion (rat)	43
Lactose	44%-64% of diet	Purified diet	$FeSO_4$	Increased versus starch or sucrose	Extrinsic (rat)	45
Lactose	44%-64% of diet	Purified diet	Reduced iron	Greater than starch Greater than sucrose	Extrinsic (rat)	45
Lactose	44%-64% of diet	Purified diet	Ferric sodium pyrophosphate	Same as starch or sucrose	Extrinsic (rat)	45
Lactose	44%-64% of diet	Purified diet	Ferric ortho phosphate	Less than sucrose and the same as starch	Extrinsic (rat)	45

Continued on next page.

Table V, continued

Chemical Added to Food	Level Added¶	Food	Iron Source	Effect of Added Chemical on Iron Bioavailability**	Test Type (species)*	Reference
Sucrose	5 g/mg Fe	Meal with radio-labeled black beans	Ferric ammonium citrate	1.8% ferric ammonium citrate 2.6% bean iron	Intrinsic Extrinsic (human)	46
Sucrose	5 g/mg Fe	Meal containing radiolabeled corn	$FeCl_3$	1.1% $FeCl_3$; 0.9% corn iron	Intrinsic Extrinsic (human)	46
Sucrose	5 g/mg Fe	Meal containing radiolabeled wheat	$FeSO_4$	3.3% $FeSO_4$; 3.0% wheat iron	Intrinsic Extrinsic (human)	47
Sucrose	5 g/mg Fe	Meal with labeled black beans	$FeSO_4$	4.3% $FeSO_4$; 3.0% wheat iron	Intrinsic Extrinsic (human)	47
Cellulose	10–30%	Bread	$FeSO_4$	No effect	Repletion (rat)	21

¶Numbers separated by a colon represent the ratio-moles of chemical added:moles of iron added.
*See Table III for explanation of test types.
**Percentages refer to the absolute percent of iron absorbed from the total dose.

corn was double that from a diet enriched with ferrous sulfate (34). In later work, the mean absorption from ferrous sulfate added to various foods varied from 2% to 30%, whereas the absorption from added NaFeEDTA remained almost unchanged (35). Some authors have advocated using NaFeEDTA as an iron fortification source in Central America, since its bioavailability is adequate and its absorption is less hampered than ferric sulfate by inhibitors in foods of the area (36).

Other organic acids which have been tested for their impact on iron absorption include oxalic, succinic, fumaric and lactic acid (Table V). The iron from iron phytates was bioavailable only in the soluble monoferric form, whereas the less soluble diand tetra-ferric phytates were very poor iron sources (37, 38). Oxalic acid may vary in its effect on iron absorption based on variation in chelate strength. Amino acids and proteins have been observed to enhance iron uptake. The effect of amino acids has been ascribed to their iron chelating property as reviewed by Forth and Rummel (48).

Carbohydrates. Several carbohydrates, particularly mono and disaccharides, have been investigated for possible effects on iron uptake (second half of Table V). Sugars which have been noted to augment iron absorption include fructose and sorbitol. These presumably act as ligands for iron with a sterically favorable attachment through hydroxy groups. Fructose has been shown effective in improving iron absorption when present in very high concentration (41, 42). A study of iron chelation by fructose and other carbohydrates determined that fructose formed the strongest complex of the sugars tested, but the complex was weak (49). Saltman hypothesized that control of iron uptake was determined by the ability of the iron to be chelated by low molecular weight ligands (50). He cited the siderosis among the Bantu of South Africa as an example of chronic iron overload due to consumption of a high concentration of iron ligands. Bantu beer, which is cooked and brewed in iron containers, may contain easily absorbed iron-sugar chelates. It was reported that fructose was a causative agent for sweet wine alcoholic's disease, a siderosis (51). Pollack et al., (41) studied fructose, glucose and galactose, all iron chelating sugars, and found that only fructose increased iron absorption (Table V). However, lactate and pyruvate, end products of fructose metabolism, also enhanced iron uptake. Reduction of ferric to the more available ferrous iron has been shown in fructose solutions (49). But sorbitol, a non-reducing sugar, also enhanced iron absorption, so reduction is not solely responsible for the effect of fructose on iron (44). Studies with lactose have shown either a decrease in iron absorption relative to sucrose (43) or an increase in absorption relative to sucrose or starch (45). The effect of lactose on iron absorption depended upon the iron source used for enrichment. For example, iron phosphates were of the same bioavailability in the presence of either lactose or starch. Glucose (41, 43), galactose (41), sucrose (46, 45, 47) and cellulose (21) all were shown to have no effect on iron absorption as shown in Table V. Iron-complexing carbohydrates, including polysaccharides and fibers, are currently being evaluated for their impact on iron chemistry and bioavailability.

Effect of Food Processing on Iron Chemistry

In many of the bioavailability studies discussed above the chemical form of iron was not known before or after processing. The question remains as to what changes may occur in the food matrix which may be responsible for observed changes in bioavailability. Some studies which examined chemical changes in iron due to processing are described in Table VI.

Ionic Iron. It was once believed that only iron which could be liberated in an ionic form from foods was bioavailable (5). This stems from the work of Elvehjem in 1932 which observed that "all iron compounds must be broken down into inorganic salts before the iron can be assimilated" (52). Not until the development of radioiron techniques was the value of chelated forms of iron, most notably the heme iron pool, fully recognized. This early emphasis on ionic iron as the sole determinant of iron bioavailability led to several studies which equated "available" iron with ionizable iron. The term "bioavailability" was first used in 1971 to distinguish available iron measured by chemical assay from (bio)available iron measured by bioassay (9). Most early studies on chemical availability of iron employed a modification of Hill's 1930 procedure using a ferrous-specific iron chromophore, alpha, alpha-dipyridyl (53). It is interesting that some of these studies were successful in correlating ionizable with bioavailable iron. In a 1942 study (54), ionizable iron agreed with bioavailable iron (as determined by heme repletion of rats) for canned frozen asparagus, green beans, lima beans and red sea perch, but not for spinach (Table VI). The authors attribute this exception to the cathartic action of spinach on the rats, as well as an interference with the chemical method. An attempt to use dipyridyl to determine ferrous iron in an artificial gastric digest was unsuccessful (55). Later work had shown ionizable iron in enriched bread was in the ferric state, but the iron source used in enrichment was not specified (56). Hodson used dipyridyl to show that ferric ortho phosphate was converted to the ferrous form after processing and storage of a canned beverage (57). More recently, the percent ionizable iron at pH 7.5 was correlated with percent iron absorbed by men (58). This was proposed as an in vitro method for measuring bioavailability of nonheme iron. A study using the bathophenanthroline reagent

Table VI. Studies which examined chemical changes in iron due to processing.

Form of iron Measured	Food	Processing	Bioavailability	Iron Source	Major Result	Reference
Ionizable	Vegetables	Canning Freezing	Repletion (rat)	Edogenous	Ionic iron agreed with heme repletion	54
Ionic (ferric only)	Bread	Baking	Not measured	Not specified	Iron in bread was in ferric state by indirect analysis	56
Ionic FeII & FeIII	Canned liquid dietaries	Retort & storage	Not measured	Ferric ortho phosphate	Mostly dissolved and in FeIII form at 2-5 months	57
Ionizable	Cereal, pulses & vegetables	Cooked	Extrinsic (men)	Endogenous	% ionizable at pH 7.5 correlated with % absorption	58
Valencies FeII, FeIII, Fe	Model systems, fruit juices & biscuit dough	pH varied	Not measured	Several sources*	Lower pH favored ferrous iron, ascorbic acid aided ionization at all pH values	59
Soluble	Beer	Brewing	Extrinsic (human)	$FeCl_3$	Brewing lowered pH and increased bioavailability, but absorption from beer exceeded gruel at same pH	26
Soluble	Various foods	*in vitro* gastric	Not measured	Endogenous	Chemically available iron agrees with bioavailability as determined by (32)	60
Soluble	Enriched soda crackers	Baking	Repletion from simulated digest (rat)	$FeSO_4$ H_2 reduced	Increased pH & less solubility with no change in bioavaiability	20
Soluble	Cured beef	Smoked & cooked	Repletion (rat)	Endogenous	Both bioavailability and soluble iron decreased as nitrite increased	6

Continued on next page.

Table VI, continued

Form of iron Measured	Food	Processing	Bioavailability	Iron Source	Major Result	Reference
Iron profile#	Ascorbic acid beverage	Freeze dry	Not measured	Several sources*	No changes in iron profile	61
Iron profile#	Ascorbic acid beverage	Spray dry	Not measured	Several sources*	Ferrous iron formed depending upon iron source added	61
Iron profile#	Baking soda biscuits	Baking	Not measured	Several sources*	Mostly insoluble after baking, similar profile to commercial breads	62
Iron profile#	Canned spinach puree	Retort	Not measured	Several sources*	Insoluble and ferrous increased, ascorbic acid favored ferrous form, FeEDTA minimally affected	64
Iron profile#	Canned liquid milk product	Retort	Repletion (rat)	Ferric ortho phosphate	Bioavailability unchanged; no soluble iron detected	15
Iron profile#	Canned liquid milk product	Retort	Repletion (rat)	Electrolytic	Bioavailability increased; 59% ferrous iron	15
Iron profile#	Canned liquid milk product	Retort	Repletion (rat)	Carbonyl	Bioavailability increased; 59% ferrous iron	15
Iron profile#	Canned liquid milk product	Retort & 6 or 12 months storage	Repletion (rat)	Ferric ortho phosphate	Bioavailability very low; only insoluble iron detected	65
Iron profile#	Canned liquid milk product	Retort & 6 or 12 months storage	Repletion (rat)	Electrolytic	High bioavailability and ferrous formed (Table IX)	65

Form of iron Measured	Food	Processing	Bioavailability	Iron Source	Major Result	Reference
Iron profile#	Canned liquid milk	Retort & 6 or 12 months storage	Repletion (rat)	Carbonyl	High bioavailability and ferrous formed (Table IX)	65

*Several iron sources include: ferrous sulfate, ferric ortho phosphate, sodium ferric EDTA, H_2 reduced iron, electrolytic iron, carbonly iron and endogenous iron.

#The iron profile measures the ferrous (FeII), ferric (FeIII) and elemental (Fe) iron valencies, as well as soluble, complexed and total iron.

to measure iron valence had shown that ferrous was favored in foods or model systems at low pH values (59). These data are discussed in the chapter on physiochemical properties in this book. Of interest is that at pH 6.2 (approximate duodenal pH) precipitation of ferric hydroxides required 2 to 7 days. This has significance for the absorption of ionic iron even in the absence of chelators which aid solubility at high pH values.

Soluble Iron. Some researchers have measured soluble or water-extractable iron from foods with varying degrees of agreement with bioavailability data. These studies are also listed in Table VI. Fox and Bender (60) reported that chemically available iron resulting from the action of human gastric juice on several foods agreed with bioavailability as reported by Layrisse et al. (25). Compared to bread, cracker manufacture increased pH and reduced solubility of iron under simulated gastric conditions, with no change in bioavailability (20). A decrease in bioavailability from 58% to 39% with a corresponding decrease in water-extractable iron from 8.7 to 2.6 mg/kg was observed in cured beef as the nitrite content increased from 0 to 50 ppm (44). Curiously, above 50 ppm nitrite, bioavailability increased with little change in extractable iron. The process of brewing corn-sorgum beer (which included a lactic acid-generating fermentation) increased solubility as well as bioavailability of iron (26). However, the absorption from beer was still greater than absorption from an iron solution at the same pH as the beer.

Iron Profile. The studies reviewed in the section on the effect of processing on iron bioavailability suggest that bioavailability depends upon the iron source, the food matrix, and the nature of the food process. The question remains does the source, matrix or the process have an effect on the chemical form of iron, or iron profile.

The effect of varying the source, matrix or process on the chemical form of iron was determined in a series of studies by this author (end of Table VI). Several iron sources were added to a pH 3.5 ascorbic acid-fortified beverage which contained sucrose and citric acid (61). Changes in ionic (ferrous plus ferric) iron were followed over 3 to 4 days without further processing (Figure 1). Added iron changed in chemical form, depending upon the identity of the iron source added; ferrous sulfate remained in the ferrous form; ferric ortho phosphate, although a very insoluble iron source, was 17% ionic at 3 days; ferric EDTA remained complexed with only 4 to 7% ionic iron, and H_2 reduced iron was rapidly oxidized to ferrous iron. Ionic iron remaining after spray drying without any storage period is shown as the unconnected points on the right of Figure 1. Spray drying caused the same changes as storage, but some conversion

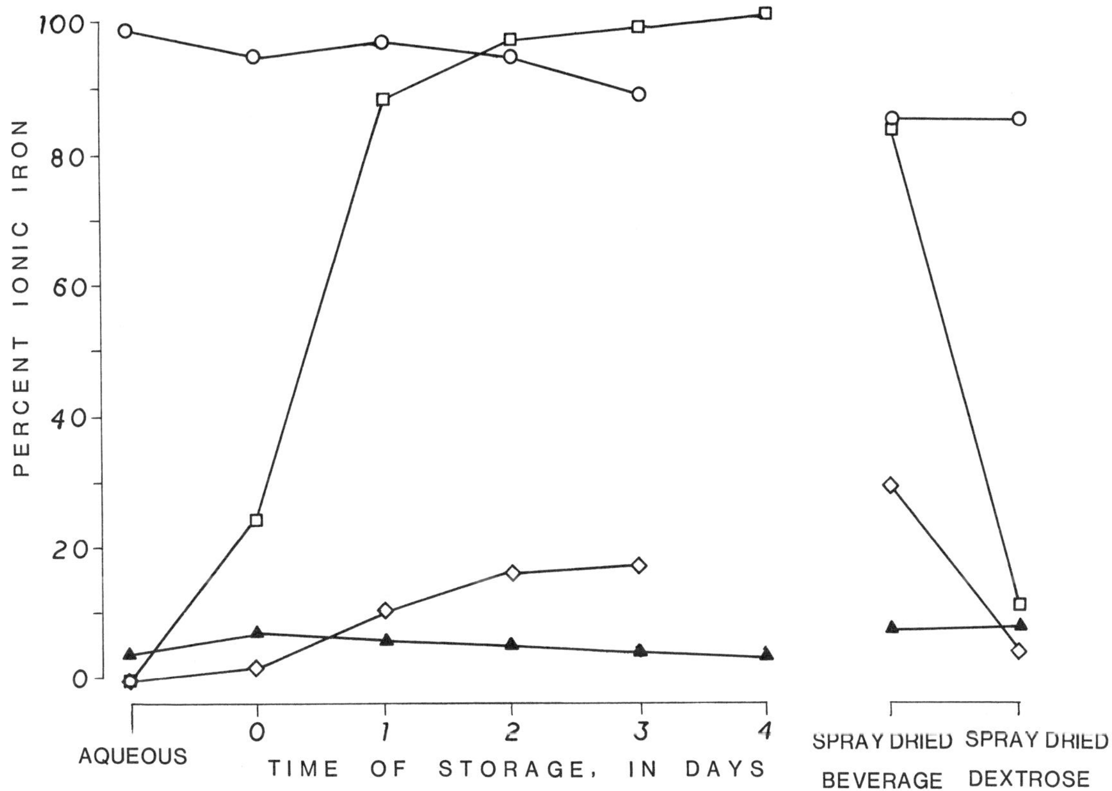

Figure 1. The effect of storage and spray drying on the ionic (ferrous and ferric) iron in a vitamin C-enriched beverage. The amount of ionic iron depended upon the iron source added to the beverage. Little change took place when the beverage was replaced by a dextrose solution (compare far left and far right sets of points). Iron key: ○, ferrous sulfate; □, elemental iron; ◇, ferric orthophosphate; ▲, ferric sodium EDTA.

of ferrous sulfate and H_2 reduced iron to ferric and complexed forms took place (not shown). The effect of spray drying alone, without the beverage matrix, was examined by drying each iron source in a dextrose solution. These data are plotted on the far right of Figure 1. Practically no differences were observed relative to aqueous controls, illustrating the importance of the beverage matrix in determining the form of iron after processing.

Freeze drying (not shown) was shown to have no effect on the 4 iron sources tested, but did alter a solution of heme iron. After freeze drying, only 54% of the original heme complex remained, with nearly all remaining iron in the ferrous form. Mahoney et al. reported oxidation of freeze dried beef decreased the bioavailability of the iron (6). It is possible that the beef iron was chemically modified.

Another dry-heat process, baking of baking soda biscuits, provided a high pH matrix (62). Baking favored insoluble iron for all iron sources baked into biscuits. The greatest amount of insoluble iron resulted when ferric ortho phosphate was added, the least when NaFeEDTA was added. About half of NaFeEDTA remained in the complexed form after baking. Based on these findings and the bioavailability data in the previous section, NaFeEDTA may be appropriate for enriched baked goods. The final form of iron depended upon the iron source added prior to baking, analogous to what was observed in feeding studies. Ferrous sulfate enriched biscuits had the most ionic iron after baking. Elemental iron sources retained from 10 to 22% of the original elemental form after baking. This may have significance as elemental iron in the presence of hydrochloric acid oxidizes to the soluble ferrous form (63). Commercially produced yeast-leavened breads were also profiled. Ferrous sulfate enriched bread had a large amount of complexed iron present. Work in progress should shed more light on the nature of the complexed iron in grains and cereals.

The effect of a wet-heat process, thermal processing in glass, was studied using a spinach puree (64). Spinach contains a large amount of endogenous iron, 3 to 5 mg per 100 grams, but the bioavailability of this iron was shown to be both poor and good by different labs (25, 39). Poor bioavailability of spinach iron has been attributed to binding by endogenous oxalic acid or phosphates which render it insoluble and unabsorbable (4). The presence of insoluble iron was verified (Table VII). Endogenous iron in raw, thermally processed, and commercial samples of canned spinach was from 96% (raw) to 85% (cooked) insoluble (64). Thermal processing increased the ferrous iron in spinach from baseline levels to 11% (Table VII). Increased ferrous iron occurred in all samples to which iron was added before processing, except heme iron which was insoluble. Heme may have been exceptional due to insolubility at low pH values. Sodium ferric pyrophosphate increased from 1 to 24% ferrous

Table VII. Ferrous iron recovered from raw and processed spinach with and without added iron sources.

Added iron Source	% Ferrous Iron		
	Before Process	After Process	After Process with Ascorbate
None (endogenous iron)	nd	11	5
Ferrous sulfate	5	24	19
Ferric ortho phosphate	nd	2	12
Ferric sodium pyrophosphate	1	24	24
Ferric sodium EDTA	nd	3	13
Heme (methemoglobin)	11	2	1
H2 reduced iron	7	12	27
Electrolytic	5	14	24
Carbonyl	6	17	25

after processing. This may help explain the enhanced bioavailability observed by some authors with this iron source. Adding ascorbic acid increased ferrous iron to higher levels after processing, with the exception of heme, ferrous sulfate and endogenous iron. Oxidation reduction potentials were highest (least reducing) for the three exceptions (64). In this matrix, ascorbic acid appeared to function as a reducing agent rather than a chelator.

Agreement between iron profile and bioavailability data was observed for a retort processed canned milk product (15, 65). Clemens and Mercurio (15) reported a large increase in bioavailability (by rat heme repletion) for electrolytic and carbonyl iron, but not for ferric ortho phosphate after processing (Study 1 in Table VIII). The iron profile revealed that ferric ortho phosphate was insoluble, whereas electrolytic and carbonyl iron samples both contained 59% ferrous iron after process. In a later study (study 2 in Table VIII), these products were analyzed after 6 to 12 months storage (65). Bioavailability of ferric ortho phosphate remained very low and its iron profile did not change. The pH of this food matrix was 6.6, which may not favor ionization of an insoluble iron source. Both elemental iron sources had lower bioavailabilities after storage than when freshly processed, corresponding to less ferrous and less soluble iron. Changes in bioavailability correlated with changes in ionic, ferrous and soluble iron. The relationship appeared to be geometric as shown in Figure 2, a plot of % ionic

Table VIII. Iron profiles and bioavailability, processed and stored canned liquid milk-based products

Iron Source and Treatment	RBV[1]		Valence Profile, %			Solubility Profile		
	Study 1	Study 2	Fe°	FeII	FeIII	Soluble	Insoluble	Complexed
Ferric ortho phosphate								
Unprocessed	24							
Processed	-14		1	nd	nd	nd	100	nd
Processed with 6 months storage		31	1	nd	nd	nd	100	nd
Processed with 12 months storage		19	nd	nd	nd	nd	100	nd
Electrolytic iron								
Unprocessed	123							
Processed	297		nd	59	5	71	29	7
Processed & 6 months storage		90	2	42	1	42	58	nd
Processed & 12 months storage		107	nd	40	2	47	53	3
Carbonyl iron								
Unprocessed	66							
Processed	202		1	59	3	70	30	9
Processed & 6 months storage		119	1	39	2	41	59	nd
Processed & 12 months storage		69	nd	23	3	33	67	6

[1]RBV = relative biological value, where a reference dose of ferrous sulfate = 100.
nd = not detected.

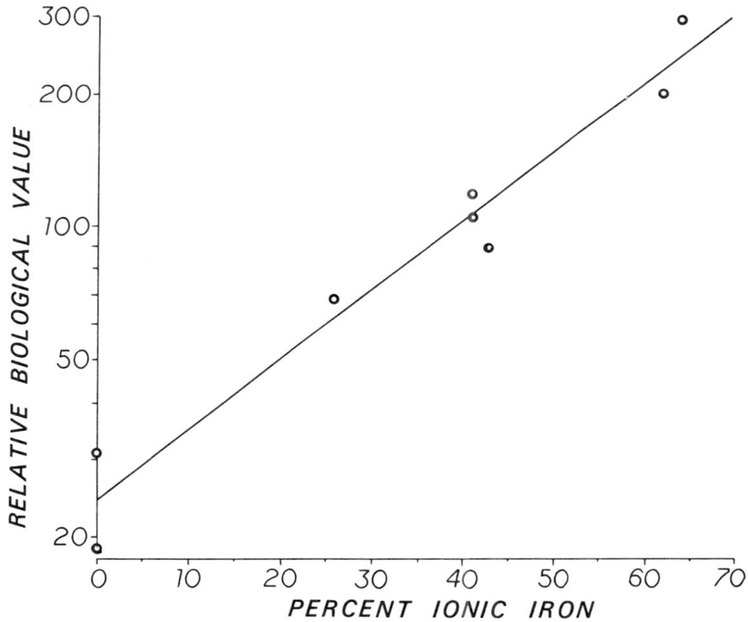

Figure 2. Chemical and biological changes in iron observed after retort-processing a milk-based beverage (47, 90). As the percent of ionic iron increased, the relative biological value in rats increased geometrically.

iron versus bioavailability. For these data, ionic iron may be useful as a predictor of bioavailability for some foods. This agrees with earlier work which proposed ionizable iron as an *in vitro* test for bioavailability (58).

More data are needed in order to determine the exact relationship between chemical forms of iron and bioavailability. However, it appears hopeful that simple chemical measures may soon be available to estimate iron bioavailability for a particular food and process.

Literature Cited

1. Spiro, T. G.; Saltman, P. "Iron in Biochemistry and Medicine"; Inorganic Chemistry. A. Jacobs and M. Worwood, Eds.; Academic Press: New York, 1974; p 1-26.
2. Lee, K.; Clydesdale, F. M. *CRC Critic. Rev. Food Sci. Nutr.* 1979, *11*, (2), 117-153.
3. Livingston, D. J.; Brown, W. D. *Food Technol.* 1981, *35*, (5), 244.
4. Forth, W.; Rummel, W. *Physiol. Rev.* 1973, *53*, 724-792.
5. Waddell, J. Life Sciences Research Office, FASEB: Bethesda, MD, 1973.
6. Mahoney, A. W.; Hendricks, D. G.; Gillett, T. A.; Buck, D. R.; Miller, C. G. *J. Nutr.* 1979, *109*, 2182-2189.
7. Bass, E. J.; Borenstein, B.; Brooke, C. L.; Gortner, W. A.; O'Neill, R. D.; Rusoff, I.; Titus, D.; Bandle, M. R. American Bakers Association: Washington, D.C.; Millers' National Federation: Chicago, IL, 1972.
8. Fritz, J. C.; Pla, G. W.; Rollinson, C. L. *Bakers Digest* 1975, *49*, (2), 46-49.
9. Pla, G. W.; Fritz, J. C. *J. Assoc. Off. Anal. Chem.* 1971, *54*, 13.
10. Fritz, J. C.; Pla, G. W. *J. Assoc. Off. Anal. Chem.* 1972, *55*, 1129-1137.
11. Fritz, J. C.; Pla, G. W.; Harrison, B. N.; Clark, G. A. *J. Assoc. Off. Anal. Chem.* 1974, *57*, 513-517.
12. Fritz, J. C.; Pla, G. W.; Harrison, B. N.; Clark, G. A.; Smith, E. A. *J. Assoc. Off. Anal. Chem.* 1978, *61*, 709-14.
13. Theuer, R. C.; Kemmerer, K. S.; Martin, W. H.; Zoumas, B. L.; Sarett, H. P. *J. Agr. Food Chem.* 1971, *19*, 555-558.
14. Theuer, R. C.; Martin, W. H.; Wallander, J. F.; Sarett, H. P. *J. Agr. Food Chem.* 1973, *21*, 482-485.
15. Clemens, R. A.; Mercurio, K. C. *J. Food Sci.* 1981, *46*, 930-932.
16. Coccodrilli, G. D.; Reussner, G. H.; Thiessen, R. *J. Agr. Food Chem.* 1976, *24*, 351-353.
17. Cook, J. D.; Minnich, V.; Moore, C. V.; Rasmussen, A.; Bradley, W. B.; Finch, C. A. *Am. J. Clin. Nutr.* 1973, *26*, 861-872.

18. Callender, S. T.; Warner, G. T. Am. J. Clin. Nutr. 1968, 21, 1170-1174.
19. Disler, P. B.; Lynch, S. R.; Charlton, R. W.; Bothwell, T. H. Br. J. Nutr. 1975, 34, 141-152.
20. Ranhotra, G. S.; Loewe, R. J.; Puyat, L. V. Cereal Chem. 1973, 50, 745-749.
21. Ranhotra, G. S.; Lee, C.; Gelroth, J. A. Nutr. Rep. Int. 1979, 19, 851-857.
22. Rees, J. M.; Monsen, E. R. J. Agr. Food Chem. 1973, 21, 913-915.
23. Wood, R. J.; Stake, P. E.; Eiseman, J. H.; Shippee, R. L.; Wolski, K. E.; Koehn, U. J. Nutr. 1979, 108, 1477-1484.
24. Sayers, M. H.; Lynch, S. R.; Jacobs, P.; Carlton, R. W.; Bothwell, T. H.; Walker, R. B.; Mayet, F. Br. J. Hematol. 1973, 24, 209-218.
25. Layrisse, M.; Cook, J. D.; Martinez, C.; Roche, M., Kuhn, I. N.; Walker, R. B.; Finch, C. A. Blood. 1969, 33, 530-543.
26. Derman, D. P.; Bothwell, T. H.; Torrance, J. D.; Bezwoda, R. W.; MacPhail, A. P.; Kew, M. C.; Sayers, M. H.; Disler, P. B.; Charlton, R. W. Br. J. Nutr. 1980, 43, 271-279.
27. Rotruck, J. T.; Luhrsen, K. R. J. Agr. Food Chem. 1979, 27, 27-33.
28. Cook, J. D.; Morck, T. A.; Lynch, S. R. Am. J. Clin. Nutr. 1981, 34, 2622-2629.
29. Cook, J. D.; Monsen, E. R. Am. J. Clin. Nutr. 1977, 30, 235-241.
30. Derman, D.; Sayers, M.; Lynch, S. R.; Charlton, R. W.; Bothwell, T. H. Br. J. Nutr. 1977, 38, 261-269.
31. Brise, H.; Hallberg, L. Acta Medica Scand. Stockholm 1962, 171, 51-54.
32. Conrad, M. E.; Schade, S. G. Gastroenterology 1968, 55, 35-45.
33. Cook, J. D.; Monsen, E. R. Am. J. Clin. Nutr. 1967, 29, 614-620.
34. Layrisse, M.; Martinez-Torres, C. Am. J. Clin. Nutr. 1977, 30, 1166-1174.
35. Martinez-Torres, C.; Romano, E. L.; Renzi, M.; Layrisse, M. Am. J. Clin. Nutr. 1979, 32, 809-816.
36. Viteri, F. E.; Garcia-Ibanez, R.; Torun, B. Am. J. Clin. Nutr. 1978, 31, 961-971.
37. Ellis, R.; Morris, E. R. Nutr. Rep. Int. 1979, 20, (5), 739-747.
38. Lipshitz, D. A.; Simpson, K. M.; Cook, J. D.; Morris, E. R. J. Nutr. 1979, 109, 1154-1160.
39. Van Campen, D. R.; Welch, R. M. J. Nutr. 1980, 110, 1618.
40. Brise, H.; Hallberg, L. Acta Medica Scan.: Stockholm. 1962, 171, 23-27.
41. Pollack, S.; Kaufman, R. M.; Crosby, W. H. Blood. 1964, 24, 577-581.

42. Pollycove, M.; Saltman, P.; Fish, M.; Newman, R.; Tono, M. Clin. Res. 1972, 20, 183.
43. Pennell, M. D.; Davies, M. I.; Rasper, J.; Motzok, I. J. Nutr. 1976, 106, 265-274.
44. Loria, A.; Medal, L. S.; Elizondo, J. Am. J. Clin. Nutr. 1962, 10, 124-127.
45. Amine, E. K.; Hegsted, D. M. J. Agr. Food Chem. 1975, 23, 203-208.
46. Layrisse, M.; Martinez-Torres, C.; Renzi, M.; Velez, F.; Gonzalez, M. Am. J. Clin. Nutr. 1976, 29, 8-18.
47. Layrisse, M.; Martinez-Torres, C.; Renzi, M. Am. J. Clin. Nutr. 1976, 29, 274-279.
48. Davis, P. S.; Deller, D. J. Austral. Annals Med. 1967, 16, (1), 70-74.
49. Kearsley, M. W.; Birch, G. G. Food Chem. 1976, 2, 209-17.
50. Saltman, P. J. Chem. Ed. 1965, 42, 682-687.
51. Saltman, P.; Hegenauer, J.; Christopher, J. Annals Clin. Lab. Sci. 1976, 6, 167.
52. Elvehjem, C. A. J. Biol. Chem. 1930, 86, 463-467.
53. Hill, R. Royal Soc. London Proc. 1930, 107, 205-214.
54. Theriault, F. R.; Fellers. Food Res. 1942, 7, 503-508.
55. Kirch, E. R.; Bergeim, O.; Kleinberg, J.; and James, S. J. Biol. Chem. 1947, 171, 687-694.
56. Leichter, J.; Joslyn, M. A. Cereal Chem. 1967, 44, 346-52.
57. Hodson, A. Z. J. Agr. Food Chem. 1970, 18, 946-947.
58. Narasinga-Rao, B. S.; Prabhavathi, T. Am. J. Clin. Nutr. 1978, 31, 169-175.
59. Nojeim, S. J.; Clydesdale, F. M. J. Food Sci. 1981, 46, 606-611.
60. Fox, S. J.; Bender, A. E. Proc. Nutr. Soc. 1978, 37, 61A.
61. Lee, K.; Clydesdale, F. M. J. Food Sci. 1980, 45, 711-15.
62. Lee, K.; Clydesdale, F. M. J. Food Sci. 1980, 45, 1500.
63. Lee, K. Unpublished data.
64. Lee, K.; Clydesdale, F. M. J. Food Sci. 1981, 46, 1064-68.
65. Clemens, R. A. J. Food Sci. 1981, 47, 228-230.
66. Forth, W.; Rummel, W. "Intern. Encyclop. Pharmacology and Therapeutics", Vol. I and II, Pergamon Press, 1975; p 599.

RECEIVED June 2, 1982.

4

The Effects of Physicochemical Properties of Food on the Chemical Status of Iron

F. M. CLYDESDALE

University of Massachusetts, Department of Food Science and Nutrition, Amherst, MA 01003

Iron bioavailability is affected by valence state, form, solubility, particle size, and complexation which in turn may be affected by the food matrix. Complexation of iron has been found to have either a positive or negative effect on availability, with such compounds as ascorbic acid and fructose increasing availability and oxalates, phytates, phosphates and food fibers perhaps decreasing availability. Availability has also been shown to be directly correlated to acid solubility. We have found that acidity tends to increase ionization as well as favoring the ferrous state which has greater solubility at the pH of the intestine (10^{-1}M) than does ferric (10^{-18}M). Both reduction potential and dissolved oxygen may also affect ionization and valence state with the former having the most potent effect from results we obtained.

These factors, which are inherent in the food system, must be considered if the problems of iron deficiency are to be combatted successfully.

0097-6156/82/0203-0055$08.50/0

The 1977-78 Nationwide Food Consumption Survey (NFCS) recently published by the USDA (1) outlines the following findings as related to iron intake in the U.S.:

1. Average iron intakes of females 12 to 50 years were 35% and 40% below the RDA, as in 1965.
2. The iron intake of infants in 1977 was more than twice the intake in 1965. However, the average intake of 1 to 2 year olds was much lower, about 45% below the 1974 RDA.

These findings were an exception to the general trend which indicated that food used by households in 1977 had a higher nutrient density than food used in 1965 and were in fact related to specific sex/age groups. Nevertheless, it is apparent that problems still exist with iron nutriture in the U.S., certainly in part due to the form of iron in the diet and what it is eaten with, rather than the total quantity of iron in the diet.

From these results it would seem logical that research must be aimed at a better understanding of not only the exact mode of action of iron absorption but also an understanding of the factors which produce and maintain the most bioavailable forms of iron in food.

This paper will attempt to address this latter point by discussing some of the physicochemical properties of food which may effect the chemical status of iron. Obviously not every property may be considered and therefore this discussion will be limited to a consideration of selected complexes, pH, and reduction potential.

Iron within a food matrix provides an extremely reactive vehicle for complexation with a great number of chemical compounds. In fact, it is this very reactivity which makes some of the most bioavailable forms of iron so objectionable to the food processor since the chemical reactions which occur can drastically affect quality. Conversely, the most functionally suitable forms of iron are often not very bioavailable. This nutritional/functional compatability, although not a subject of focus here, should be mentioned since any fortification program must consider this compatability factor or it will be doomed to failure. This problem has been discussed in some detail by Lee and Clydesdale (2) and Zoller *et al* (3).

Saltman (4) in discussing bioavailability has stated that "In essence the regulation and control of iron metabolism through the intestine as well as across all biological membranes is determined by the ability of the iron to be chelated by low molecular weight ligands". Whether or not this is an overstatement remains to be seen, but nevertheless it points out the potential role of ligands in iron chemistry both in humans and in food. The factor which probably contributes most to the potential biological role of ligands in food is their effect on iron solubility. Ferrous and ferric ions in solution do not occur in the free state, but are hydrated as $Fe(H_2O)_6^{+3}$ and $Fe(H_2O)_6^{+2}$ in acid and lose protons as the pH is raised to form the corresponding hydroxides ($FE(OH)_2$ and $FE(OH)_3$) in neutral and alkaline solutions [5]. These hydroxides are increasingly less soluble than their respective hydrates and in the absence of ligands, at physiological pH, the solubility of the two forms is 10^{-1} M (+2) and 10^{-16} M (+3). These solubility values however can be altered dramatically by any number of ligands in food such as proteins, amino acids, carboxylic acids, polyols and phosphates, which in turn might affect bioavailability either positively or negatively since a variety of studies have shown that biological systems seem to utilize iron better if it is in a soluble form. Therefore, ligands which form more soluble complexes might tend to increase bioavailability while those which form more insoluble complexes might have the opposite effect. Saltman et al [6] cites instances where soluble polymers such as ferric fructose and ferric citrate have been used to demonstrate massive deposition of iron in tissues of mice, rats, guinea pigs, rabbits, and other animals. Further these workers show a typical uptake pattern for ferric fructose and ferrous sulfate in guinea pigs whereby ferric fructose is retained at higher levels than ferrous sulfate, indicating greater absorption (Figure 1). They explain the pattern shown in Figure 1 on the solubility as well as separating the kinetics of iron absorption into three phases. During the first phase, there is very rapid excretion of the unabsorbed iron via the feces, owing in part to the formation of unabsorbable precipitates of iron polymer in the intestinal lumen. During the second phase, mucosal tissue, which has stored but not transported iron, is slowly sloughed off and is excreted. In the third, iron enters the bloodstream and circulates to the tissue where it remains until it is mobilized by normal turnover or biological demand. However, it should be recognized that although the efficacy of iron fructose complexes has been shown by several workers [7, 8] evidence to the contrary has been presented by Heinrich et al [9] who studied the effect of large amounts of fructose on therapeutic doses of ferric and ferrous iron in man and found no differences in absorption. Further, it should be recognized that reduction of ferric iron into the more soluble ferrous iron can occur in fructose solutions [8] which must be taken into account in any explanation of increased bioavailability. However, since sorbitol, a non-reducing sugar, has been found to enhance iron absorption [10] it must be concluded that the complexation of iron and not solely valence or solubility affects absorption.

The general phenomenon of carbohydrate-metal complexing is well known with a review having been written some years ago [11] and extensive research having been conducted since that time. Some studies have indicated a slight improvement in absorption from lactose and sucrose and a decrease due to starch [12] with glucose [7] having no effect.

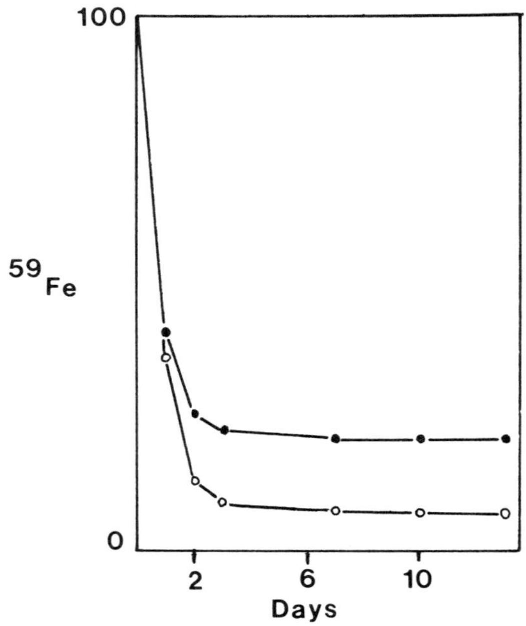

Figure 1. Kinetic pattern of ^{59}Fe retention by a guinea pig given a single initial dose of isotope per os. Key: ●, ferric fructose; ○, ferrous sulfate. (Reproduced, with permission, from Ref. 6. Copyright 1976, Institute for Clinical Nutrition.)

The differences in bioavailability found with certain complexes from study to study are frustrating at best. It seems difficult to isolate the exact affect of a given ligand and the particular complex it might form. For instance, Derman *et al* (13) recently found that iron absorption from maize and sorghum beer was more than twelve-fold greater than from a gruel made from the constituents used to prepare the beer. The authors postulated that at least three factors are responsible for this: 1) the removal of solids during fermentation, 2) the presence of ethanol, and 3) the presence of lactic acid. However, to suggest a particular ligand to explain this effect would be almost impossible.

The difficulty is also probably due in part to the chemistry involved. Bachran and Bernhard (14) reported the formation of a soluble lactose . $FeCl_2$ complex along with a precipitate of a lactose-iron gel, an insoluble lactose . $Fe(OH)_2$ adduct and insoluble $Fe(OH)_2$. The amount of each of these forms was found to vary in this work which was based on carefully controlled model systems, therefore, it would not be very surprising to find tremendous variation in food materials where conditions are subject to the vagaries of nature. Such variations would directly affect the amount of soluble and insoluble complexes, and perhaps the strength of the chelating bonds, both of which would affect the bioavailability.

Other carbohydrates which act as ligands are included in that diffuse classification of materials known as dietary fiber. Although all dietary fibers are not carbohydrates, it seems advantageous to discuss them as a group, since they are generally treated in that manner. The literature is literally bulging with reports on the bioavailability of iron from plant materials. In general, it has been found that both intrinsic and added iron in vegetables is less available than in other sources as summarized by Layrisse and Martinez-Torres (15)(Figure 2). However, other research seems to provide conflicting data and a paucity of consistent explanations for either increased or decreased bioavailability. This is not a reflection of the research, but more a reflection of the complexity of the human/food/nutrient interaction chain. Although many chemical constituents are involved, such as phosphorous (16), proteins (17-20), phytates, which have been extensively studied by Morris and Ellis of the USDA and recently by Cheryan (21), and carboxylic acids, it seems that a great deal of the binding may be due to the dietary fibers.

One component of dietary fiber, pectin, has long been known to form chelates with a number of divalent metals. Haug and Smidsrod (22) reported on the selectivity of some anionic polymers, including pectates, for divalent metal ions and Schweiger *et al* (23) have presented data in support of the formation of both intermolecular and intramolecular chelates of pectin with divalent metals. Recently Camire and Clydesdale (24) reported significant binding of iron, calcium, magnesium, and zinc by both pectin and

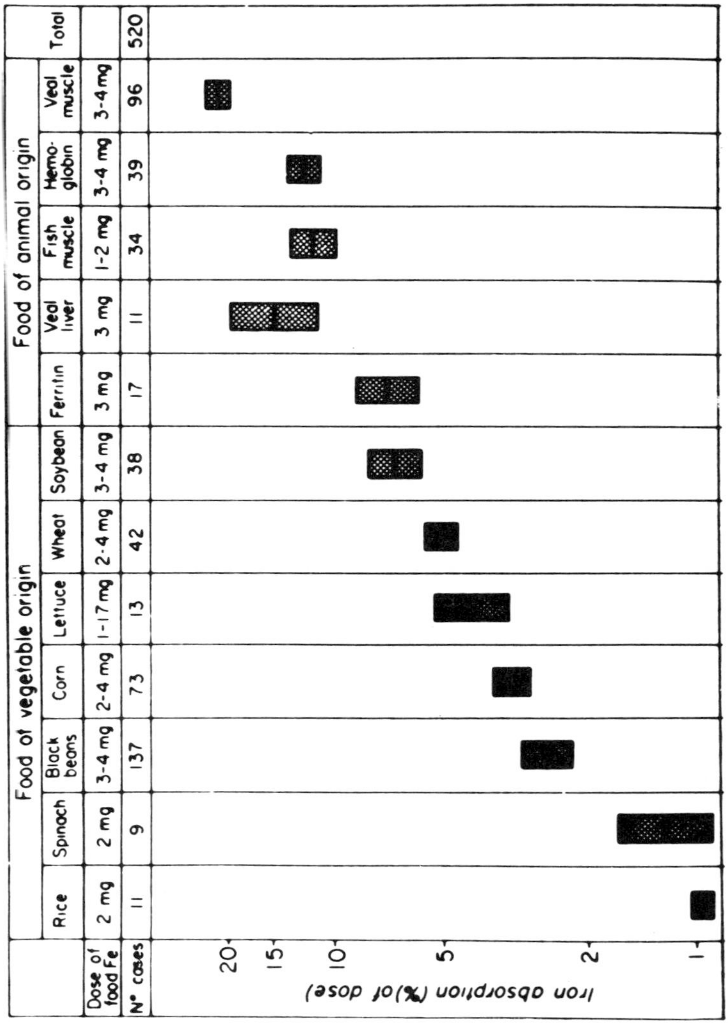

Figure 2. Iron absorption by adults from a range of foods. The bars represent the mean absorptions and standard errors, calculated from the logarithms of the percentage absorptions. (Reproduced, with permission, from Ref. 15. Copyright 1971, Grune and Stratton, Inc.)

guar gum. Barry and Halsey (25) did not find any observable binding of an extract of locust bean gum, which is a galactomannin like guar gum, with H^+, Na^+, K^+, Ag^+, Ba^{+2}, $C_2H_3O_2^-$, Cl^-, NO_3^-, SO_4^{-2}, or HSO_4^-. However, they did not investigate Fe^{+2}, Fe^{+3}, Ca^{+2}, Mg^{+2} or Zn^{+2}.

The binding of guar gum may most easily be explained by the formation of a negative charge density from contributing hydroxyl groups which exist in a sterically suitable conformation. For instance, Angyal (26) proposes that a calcium-inositol complex (neutral polysaccharide) owes its binding to an axial-equatorial-axial arrangements of hydroxyl groups to create a negative charge density. Further he proposes that the metal ion may also bind to more than three oxygen atoms and supports this proposal by using calcium-alginate (acidic polysaccharide) as an example, whereby a calcium ion is coordinated to the axial-equatorial-axial site of one chain and a carboxylate ion of another chain causing packing of the chains and thereby gelation.

Alternatively, he suggests that it is also possible for the 3 oxygen atoms in the axial-equatorial-axial sequence from one residue to bind a metal along with the carboxylate ion and another oxygen atom of an adjacent uronic acid residue.

In order to understand the binding of cations by polyuronic acids, like pectin, Grant (27) refers to three main factors that must be considered:

1. geometry of the ligand
2. separation between unit charges on the chain
3. the ease with which the polysaccharide chains can pack.

The culmination of these conclusions has resulted in a proposal of an "egg-box" model for the mechanism of binding involving two or more polysaccharide chains. Further understanding of polyuronic acid binding may be obtained from a consideration of the observation that pectins and pectinaceous fibers have the ability to interact with dietary lipids resulting in increased excretion of fecal lipids. It has been speculated that a high degree of methoxylation, high viscosity and solubility are the critical parameters which promote this excretion of fats with the increase in methoxylation increasing the hydrophobic interaction between pectins and lipids (28). However, Nagyvary and Bradbury (29) have proposed a different potential mechanism involving minerals, the implications of which, are most pertinent to this discussion. They postulate a simple model by which acidic polysaccharides such as alginates or pectins may be converted into anion exchangers by complexing with trivalent cations such as aluminum, which have the ability to bind a variety of anions that would include fatty acids and bile acids. Their model is shown in Figure 3 where it may be seen that trivalent aluminum bound to pectate offers a bonding bridge to negatively charged anionic micelles such as bile acids and/or fatty acids. Nagyvary and Bradbury (29)postulate that this binding offers a hydrophobic region to cholesterol which may partition itself as shown in Figure 3, thus explaining their finding

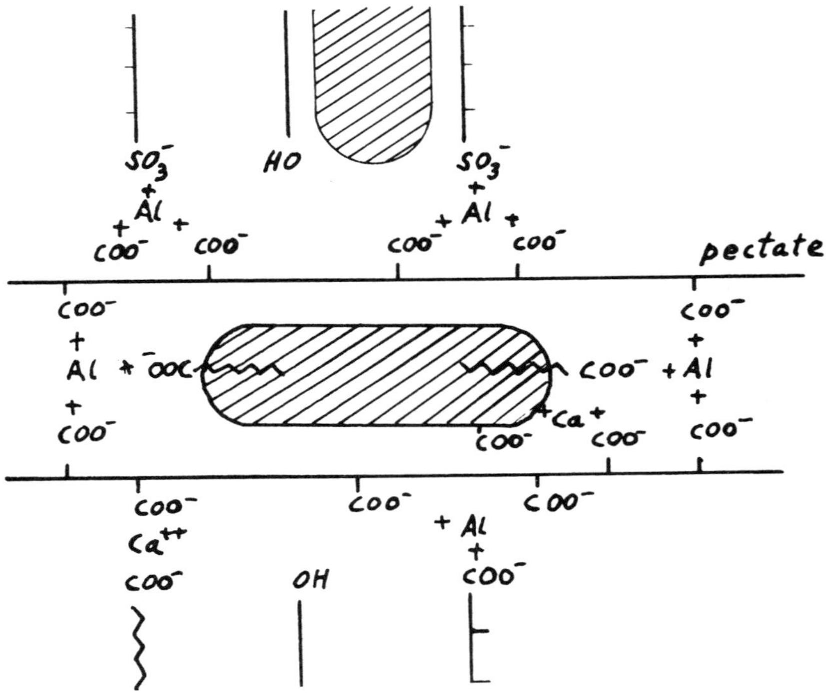

Figure 3. Hypothetical structure of a polyuronate Al^{3+} micelle complex. (Reproduced, with permission, from Ref. 29. Copyright 1977, Academic Press, Inc.)

that aluminum pectate and alginate had a strong hypocholesterolemic effect in rats.

Furda (28) examined this hypothesis by utilizing natural insoluble pectinaceous fibers in conjunction with several cations, including, H^+, Ca^{2+}, Fe^{2+}, Fe^{3+}, and Al^{3+}. If the hypothesis was correct the pectinaceous fibers bound by trivalent cations should display greater affinity for fatty acids than those neutralized by H^+ or divalent cations.

The selected fiber-cation complexes were stirred into emulsions containing fatty acids and subsequently examined. Figure 4 illustrates the results where it may be seen that the ferric-fiber complex caused a clear separation of phases apparently due to an almost quantitative interaction between ferric-fiber and fatty acids. The ferric-fiber broke the emulsion, bound virtually all the fatty acid present in the system and floated to the top thus creating a clear solution. The aluminum-fiber caused only partial separation while the H^+, Ca^{2+} and Fe^{2+} neutralized fibers did not separate or show any preference for the hydrophobic or hydrophylic phase and formed a homogeneous dispersion.

Furda (28) suggests that for steric reasons it is more likely that two carboxylic acid groups rather than three, which belong to neighboring galacturonic acid residues in the linear chain of segments of the galacturonan, can participate in binding with one trivalent cation. He suggests that this is true primarily with insoluble pectinaceous fibers. In solution (soluble pectin) the third carboxyl group could be furnished by a neighboring linear chain and result in a complete neutralization of the trivalent cation, thus inhibiting its cationic nature. If this assumption is correct, the insoluble pectinaceous fiber which has been neutralized with a trivalent cation will have a greater affinity for various anions than a fiber which has been neutralized by a divalent cation, due to a greater density of positive charge.

Furda (28) illustrates this postulation in a simplified model (Figure 5) where several hypothetical situations are shown. In the first case Fe^{2+} nearly neutralizes the fiber leaving a net positive charge of +3, in the second and third cases, Fe^{3+}, the trivalent ion produces a net positive charge of +6 and +15 respectively. He explains the greater affinity of fatty acid to the ferric-pectin complex rather than to aluminum-pectin complex by the possibility of different size cations or by the hydrophilicity of the aluminum cation, but cautions that these explanations require further research.

As important as these results may be to an understanding of the hypercholesterolemic effect which Furda discusses, we should not allow their potential significance in iron bioavailability to pass unnoticed. We would like to suggest, in fact, that such reactions could explain, in part, the seemingly greater bioavailability, often seen with ferrous iron in comparison to ferric iron. Perhaps there is a general tendency for the trivalent ion, Fe^{3+},

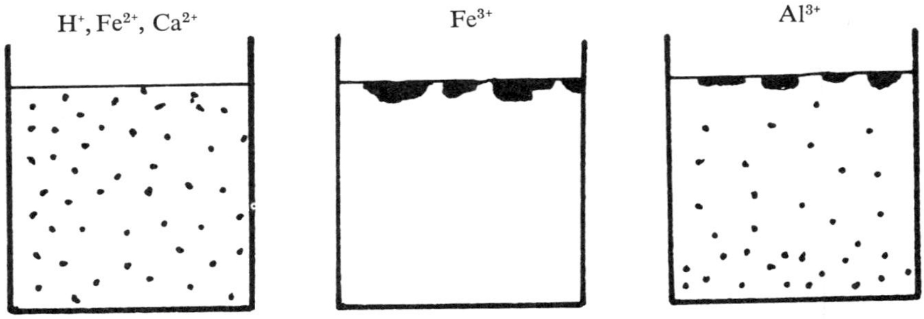

Figure 4. Interaction of pectinaceous fibers converted into different cationic forms with emulsions containing oleic acid. H^+, Fe^{2+}, Ca^{2+}—homogeneous dispersion with the emulsion having no visible phase separation; Fe^{3+}—clear separation of the fiber-oleic acid complex and the aqueous phase; Al^{3+}—heterogeneous dispersion, partial separation of phases. (Reproduced, with permission, from Ref. 28. Copyright 1979, Academic Press, Inc.)

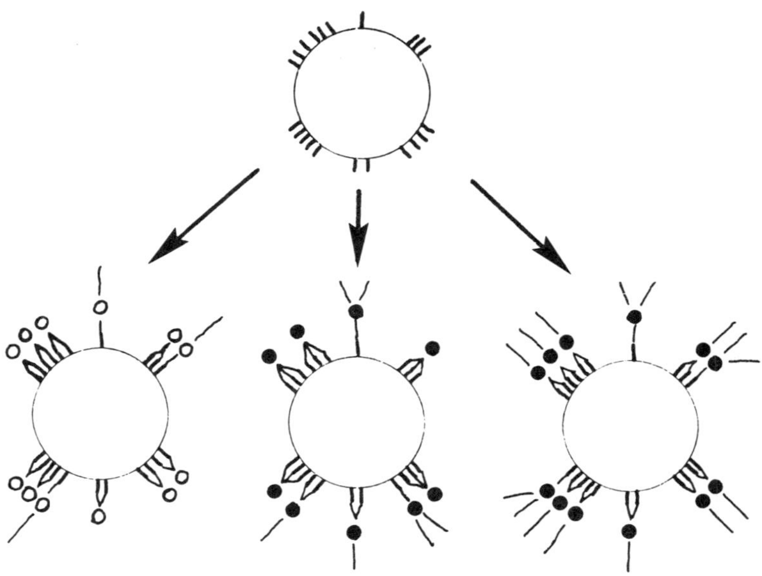

Figure 5. Simplified models of insoluble pectinaceous fiber Fe^{2+} and Fe^{3+} complexes. Key: ○, Fe^{2+}; ●, Fe^{3+}; drawn lines, free COOH groups. (Reproduced, with permission, from Ref. 28. Copyright 1979, Academic Press, Inc.)

to form cationic complexes while the divalent ion, Fe^{2+}, may tend to form neutral complexes.

Such a situation would increase the reactivity of the ferric complex, which in turn would increase its potential for further binding and decrease its potential bioavailability. Conversely, the ferrous complex, would be soluble and chemically more inert, so that its potential for biological absorption would be much greater than the more reactive ferric complex. Further such complexes might also explain, in part, the contradictory results often obtained in bioavailability studies with similar iron sources consumed with different foods. The solubility, availability and concentration of reactive compounds such as fibers, carboxylic acids, amino acids, etc. would determine if the divalent and trivalent iron complexes formed were similarly or differently charged or were uncharged. This postulation regarding the cationic nature of the iron-complex and its potential effect on bioavailability is in no way a general statement to attempt to explain iron bioavailability. It is recognized that the mechanisms for iron absorption are affected by many variables, some of which will be discussed later. However, the cationic nature and the charge density of iron complexes is one parameter which has not been considered previously to any great extent and may be a part of the many variables which affect the very complex mechanisms for iron absorption.

A great many studies have implicated other dietary fibers in mineral metabolism including Ranhotra et al (30, 31) who found the bioavailability of iron in ten commercial varieties of bread to range in RBV (relative biological value) from 32-80% and also concluded that simultaneous addition of cellulose and iron to bread does not appear to adversely affect the bioavailability of iron in bread using the hemoglobin repletion technique involving young rats. Lee and Clydesdale (32) found that baking bread produces insoluble forms of iron which are generally thought to be of inferior bioavailability and may be involved with the type of fiber(s) present as well as pH. Camire and Clydesdale (24) investigated the metal binding capacity of a standardized food grade wheat bran and several major fractions of dietary fiber, namely cellulose, lignin, pectin and guar gum, which was chosen as representative of a hemicellulose, with several minerals, including iron.

After establishing the fact that literally no binding occurred at pH levels below 5, each fiber sample was first analyzed for endogenous levels of metal from pH 5.0 to 7.0.

Iron, as ferrous sulfate, was added to each of the fibers to achieve a concentration of 5 ppm when made to 100 ml.

The mineral fiber complexes involving lignin, cellulose and wheat bran were subjected to three processes: toasting (1 hr.

@350° F, lignin 5 minutes), boiling (1 hr. in a boiling water bath), and incubation for 24 hours at 30°C which served as the control. Samples were filtered and the residue together with the filter paper was digested with concentrated HCl for 10 minutes, then cooled and filtered. The filtrates were analyzed via atomic absorption spectrophotometry (AAS)for soluble metal content.

The effects of pH on the binding of iron to various types of cellulose samples after 24 hours incubation at 30°C is shown in Table I. Carboxymethylcellulose bound as much as 70% of the ferrous iron at pH 7.0, compared to Whatman #3 filter paper which only bound 18% at pH = 7.0. Control samples of buffer and metal at each pH did not show any sign of metal hydroxide precipitation at the concentrations and temperature used in the study. The samples of pH 6.0 and 7.0 did however change to a faint yellow upon addition of iron.

Non-crystalline cellulose (Sigma Chemical Co.) bound less than 6% of the iron at pH = 5.0 after 24 hours incubation at 30°C and a toasting treatment did not significantly affect this binding. However, boiling resulted in a significant increase in binding to about 80 and 90% at pH 7 and 6 respectively.

Lignin bound more iron than cellulose at all three pH levels during incubation but toasting caused a significant decrease in the amount of iron bound. Interestingly the other metals investigated in this study showed quite different patterns of binding with lignin than did iron. For example, toasting of the lignin samples caused increased binding of zinc but had no effect on binding of calcium and magnesium as compared to the control. This observation lends credance to the fact that extrapolation of binding or availability in food from one mineral to another is very dangerous. In fact, the often repeated warnings about phytate decreasing availability of minerals in general is under a great deal of suspicion. The increased binding of zinc by lignin after toasting might be explained in part by the observation of Anderson and Clydesdale (33) that lignin concentration increased after toasting. Unfortunately this observation does not explain the results with iron, calcium or magnesium which might be better explained by bond strength and/or type of complex formed. Similar results were obtained with lignin after boiling.

The toasting treatment of wheat bran caused a highly significant increase in the amount of iron bound at all pH values. Interestingly this also was the cause for magnesium, but not for zinc and calcium which were not affected as greatly. The effect of boiling on iron binding was pH dependent with more being bound at pH 5.0 and no differences from the control seen at pH 6.0 and 7.0.

As well as the processing studies described above Camire and Clydesdale (24) also investigated the effect of a fractionation treatment on wheat bran which removed the water soluble polysaccharides, protein and starch. This treatment, as described by Anderson and Clydesdale (34) involved a 2 hour extraction of cold

Table I Percentage of total iron (ferrous sulfate) bound by different celluloses

Cellulose Source	pH 5.0	pH 6.0	pH 7.0
		Percent of total iron bound	
Carboxymethyl Cellulose	23.0 ± 1.4	63.3 ± 1.8	69.5 ± 2.1
Whatman #3 filter paper	1.1 ± 0.14	18.5 ± 0.71	13.0 ± 0.56
Solka Floc BW40 Cellulose	8.8 ± 0.28	55.3 ± 0.99	47.7 ± 0.70
Sigmacell Cellulose	5.6 ± 0.00	62.9 ± 0.14	38.3 ± 0.85

water soluble polysaccharides in 20°C, pH 7 water, followed by a 2 hour extraction of hot water soluble polysaccharides in 80°C water containing 0.01M EDTA. The residue remaining after these extractions was then subjected to a pepsin and pancreatic digestion to remove protein and starch from the samples. Examination of the mineral content of this fraction indicated that 67% of the endogenous iron was lost, 94% of the calcium, 99% of the magnesium, and 87% of the zinc. Obviously, the metals lost must have been bound to the soluble polysaccharides, starches, and/or proteins.

Iron was added to another aliquot of this fraction and it was found that the treatment resulted in a greater degree of binding at all pH values in comparison to the unfractionated wheat bran control. This was probably due to the fact that the lignin, cellulose and hemicellulose concentrations were increased as a result of the fractionation treatment and this study indicated that lignin and pectin have high metal binding capacities. The results of this study describing the binding of iron to various fibers under different conditions are summarized in Table II.

Another complexing agent which should be mentioned is oxalic acid. Oxalates are popularly thought to depress iron absorption and are often used to attempt to explain the observation by Layrisse and Martinez-Torres (15) and others that spinach is a poor source of dietary iron.

Oxalic acid is a dicarboxylic acid which crystallizes from aqueous solution as the white dihydrate with the two commonest forms in biological material being the mono and di-hydrates. It is a relatively strong acid and is moderately soluble in water. Of particular interest is the fact that it may be oxidized to carbon dioxide by ferric compounds which are in turn reduced to ferrous compounds.

Oxalic acid forms both soluble and insoluble salts with metal ions which is of particular nutritional importance. It forms soluble salts with alkali metal ions (Li, Na, K) and with iron. All other oxalates are sparingly soluble in water which would dramatically effect the bioavailability of the metal ions involved. Table III illustrates both the solubility and stability constants for a few selected metals (35). It may be seen that with calcium it forms a practically insoluble salt at neutral or alkaline pH, being soluble to the extent of 0.67 mg per 100 ml of water at pH 7.0 and 13°C. Zinc also has limited solubility (0.79 mg/100 ml, 18°) while Fe^{+2} and Fe^{+3} show solubilities of 22.0 ml/100 ml and "very soluble" respectively. These chemical facts and their effect on iron absorption have recently been substantiated in a biological sense by Van Campen and Welch (36) who investigated the availability to rats of iron from two varieties of spinach. Also they compared the absorption of iron between $FeCl_3$ and Fe-oxalate as well as the effects of adding 0.75% oxalate to the diet. They found that absorption of iron from both varieties of spinach was comparable to that from $FeCl_3$ and that the iron was equally avail-

Table II Percentage of added iron ($FeSO_4$) bound by cellulose, lignin and bran due to boiling, toasting and fractionation at pH, 5.0, 6.0, and 7.0

pH	24 hour control			boiling			toasting			fractionation
	cellulose	lignin	bran	cellulose	lignin	bran	cellulose	lignin	bran	bran
	percentage of added $FeSO_4$ bound									
5.0	5.6$\pm$0.0	87.3$\pm$1.27	20.1$\pm$4.38	15.1$\pm$1.27	** 64.8$\pm$0.0	** 39.4$\pm$0.0	12.9$\pm$0.14	** 35.8$\pm$3.11	** 93.2$\pm$2.55	** 37.5$\pm$2.4
6.0	62.9$\pm$0.14	92.1$\pm$2.40	18.3$\pm$0.14	** 84.3$\pm$2.97	** 67.5$\pm$0.14	16.1$\pm$0.42	70.6$\pm$1.98	** 56.8$\pm$0.0	** 95.7$\pm$0.14	** 33.4$\pm$0.28
7.0	38.2$\pm$0.85	84.4$\pm$7.64	12.7$\pm$0.42	** 77.9$\pm$0.71	** 65.6$\pm$1.41	21.2$\pm$4.53	35.1$\pm$1.56	** 60.7$\pm$2.00	** 84.1$\pm$0.99	** 29.9$\pm$2.12

** Significant at 1% level

Table III. Dissociation constants and solubilities of some oxalic acid salts

Description	(Stability constant K)	Solubility (mg/100 ml)
Calcium oxalate	3.0	0.67 (13°C)
Magnesium oxalate	2.76 (T=20°C, I=0.1)	70.0 (16°C)
Strontium oxalate	2.54 (18° → 0)	5.1 (18°C)
Ferrous oxalate	> 4.7 (18 → 0)	22.0
Ferric oxalate	9.4	very soluble
Zinc oxalate	4.9	0.79 (18°C)
Manganous oxalate ($2H_2O$)	3.9	3.1 (25°C)
Cobalt oxalate	4.7	insoluble
Copper oxalate	6.3	2.5 (25°C)

able from Fe-oxalate and $FeCl_3$. Also the addition of 0.75% oxalic acid to the diet did not depress iron absorption and if anything appeared to enhance iron utilization by rats.

This study seemed to be quite clear in showing that the oxalates do not seem to inhibit iron absorption. Therefore, other parameters will have to be evaluated to explain poor iron bioavailability from foods which might happen to contain oxalates.

No discussion of complexation of iron would be complete without mentioning ascorbic acid. Studies too numerous to list have clearly defined the positive effects of ascorbic acid on increasing the bioavailability of non-heme iron to both animals and humans. The interactions of Vitamin C and iron have recently been reviewed by Lynch and Cook (37). However, upon examination it would seem that the effects of ascorbic are due to factors which include, but are not limited to, complex formation.

If one was willing to accept some simplification, the most important factors involved in the efficiency of ascorbic acid in iron bioavailability might be listed as follows:

1. pH
2. complexation
3. oxidation-reduction potential

Since the effects of pH and reduction potential on iron bioavailability are to be discussed next it would seem logical to include a discussion of ascorbic acid in this section.

If one examines the following reaction,

$$Fe^{+3}\ (aq) + e^- \longrightarrow Fe^{+2}\ (aq)\ \text{(water solution, 25°C)}$$

it is found that the standard reduction potential is +770mv indicating a tendency to occur spontaneously in foods, since most foods have a standard reduction potential of 400mv or slightly less. However, if we examine the reduction half-reaction in basic solution,

$$Fe(OH)_3\ (s) + e^- \longrightarrow Fe(OH)_2\ (s) + (OH)^-$$

it is found that the standard reduction potential is -560mv indicating non-spontaneity in foods.

It is clear that pH plays a role in maintaining iron (II) in solution. Solubility of iron (II) at low pH is obviously a most important factor but the possible effect of the standard reduction potential of the Fe^{+3} redox couple at different pH values should not be overlooked. This may explain the results of Leichter and Joslyn (38), Lee and Clydesdale (39) and others who found that regardless of the source the iron found in bread and non-yeast leavened baked goods (high pH foods) respectively, was mainly in the iron (III) state and/or insoluble.

Such chemical changes will obviously effect bioavailability and perhaps explain some of the results reported. For instance, Brise and Hallberg (40) determined that 200-500 mg ascorbic acid more than tripled the bioavailability of 30 mg of iron administered as ferrous sulfate while 100 mg or less had little effect. Similarly, Cook and Monsen (41) determined that the increase in iron absorption from a semisynthetic meal was directly proportional to the amount of ascorbic acid added over a range of 25 to 1000 mg. The apparent dependency of the efficacy of ascorbic acid on concentration seems to indicate that the ascorbate either formed a complex and/or contributed to the solubility, and/or maintained the iron in the ferrous state, since the standard reduction potential for ascorbate in water is +400MV. Similar conclusions might also be drawn from Hodson (42) who found that after 2 to 5 months storage of a liquid weight control dietary with an excess of ascorbic acid, the iron added as ferrous sulfate remained in the ferrous valence whereas the iron added as ferric ortho phosphate has been solubilized, ionized and reduced to the bivalent form.

These results indicate that perhaps ascorbate may effect bioavailability more than another complexing and reducing agent such as fructose because it is also an acid.

In an attempt to clarify the chemical effects of pH and ascorbic acid on iron valence, Nojeim and Clydesdale (43) investigated model systems as well as attempting to extrapolate their findings to food materials. They used a phthalate/HCl/NaOH buffer system, since it covered a suitable pH range and did not react with added iron. Four iron sources; hydrogen reduced elemental (EI), ferrous sulfate monohydrate (FS), ferric ortho phosphate (FOP), and sodium ferric EDTA trihydrate (SFEDTA) were added to a series of buffers ranging from pH 2.2 to 6.2. As well, these same sources were evaluated at different molar levels of ascorbate, similar to those used by Brise and Hallberg (40). It was found that pH was indeed a factor in the ionization and valence of the four iron compounds evaluated. EI and FS were completely converted to ferrous ion within 48 hours at pH 4.2 and below. Ionization of FOP and SFEDTA was slower, incomplete, and resulted in less ferrous and more ferric iron. At pH 2.7, most of the ionized (soluble) iron remained in or was converted to the ferrous form over a one month storage period. The more reactive (less oxidized) iron compounds, EI and FS, remained 100% ionic (soluble) at pH 4.2 but showed some gradual oxidation to the trivalent state. These results are consistent with the discussion on redox potentials mentioned previously.

Ascorbic acid showed a rather contradictory role, at least at first glance. It seemed to promote the reduction of iron at low pH and the oxidation of iron at higher pH values. For instance, in the studies with FS and EI at pH 2.7 in the presence of ascorbate, nearly 100% of the EI and FS added was ionized and in the ferrous valence, where it remained for the duration of the study (one month). However, at pH 6.2, the presence of ascorbate greatly increased the ionization (solubilization) of both EI and FS but the newly ionized iron remained in the ferrous valence form for only 48 hours before further oxidation began to occur. In the case of EI about 50% of the ionic iron was in the ferrous valence, and 50% in the ferric state after 4 weeks. While with FS at pH 6.2, ferric hydroxide precipitates occurred without ascorbate within one week. The presence of ascorbate inhibited the formation of these hydroxides keeping most of the iron in the ionic ferric form as measured by the method of Lee and Clydesdale (39) which utilized bathophenanthroline. It is possible that the ascorbate inhibited the formation of the hydroxides by forming a complex with the ferric iron in the same manner as described by Conrad and Schade (44). If this was the case, the iron-ascorbate complex must have been disrupted by the iron-bathophenanthroline analysis, since the analysis indicated the presence of ionic ferric iron. These observations by Nojeim and Clydesdale (43) as well as other observations in the literature on the mode of action of ascorbic acid cannot be explained simply. For example, if the efficacy of ascorbic acid in iron nutriture was due solely to its role as chelating agent then it should not enhance bioavailability in almost every instance. Further confusion arises when it is noted that low pH ascorbic acid promotes the reduction of iron (45), but its presence at high pH seems to promote the oxidation of iron (43). Smith and Dunkley (46, 47) found ascorbic acid to have pro-oxidant properties in relation to oxidized flavor and lipid peroxidation in milk. They considered that these were attributable to two properties of ascorbic acid: the ability to reduce cupric copper to the cuprous form, and a specific association between ascorbic acid and copper that in some unexplained manner increases prooxidant activity.

These studies support the observed prooxidant effect of ascorbic acid at high pH (milk) in the presence of copper but not in the presence of iron.

In order to explain the effects observed by Nojeim and Clydesdale (43), I would like to propose a mechanism for the action of ascorbic acid in the presence of iron which might explain how it could act as both a reducing agent and a prooxidant as well as perhaps shedding some more light on its role in the chemistry and thus the bioavailability of iron.

This proposed mechanism is based on the interrelationship between solubility, pH, reduction potential, and chelation in a solution of iron and ascorbic acid.

At low pH, it will be remembered, Fe^{+3} and Fe^{+2} are soluble and probably exist as their respective hydrates with the standard reduction potential of $Fe^{+3}(aq) + e^- \rightarrow Fe^{+2}(aq)$ being +770mv. In the presence of ascorbate which has a standard reduction potential of +440mv the formation of Fe^{+2} will take place spontaneously (45, 48) and reaction 1 (Figure 6) will go to the right. However, at the same time, at a low pH, both a Fe^{+2} -ascorbate and a Fe^{+3} -ascorbate complex may form (44, 48), represented by reactions 2 and 4 (Figure 6). Upon addition of ferric iron to an ascorbic acid solution reaction 2 will probably take place more rapidly than reaction 1, but in time reaction 1 will predominant if the pH is maintained at a low level, as observed by Nojeim and Clydesdale (43), with the overall effect being reduction. Thus ascorbate, due to its reduction potential relative to iron at a low pH, and

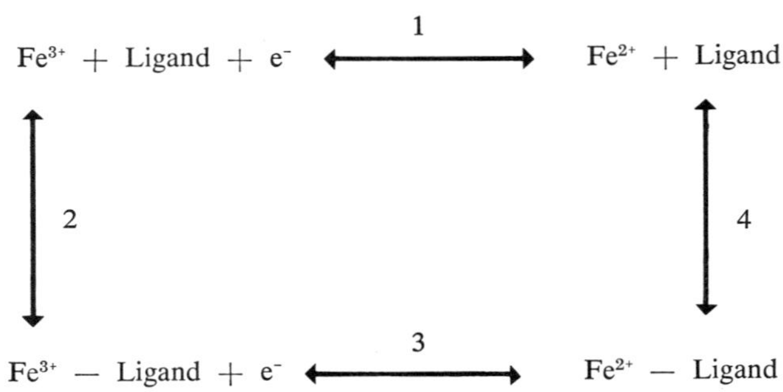

Figure 6. Interrelationship between iron (II), iron (III), and their respective ligand complexes in solution.

its ability to de-complex will act as a reducing agent with time. This implies that with time in an acid solution containing Fe^{+3} and ascorbate that the Fe^{+2} form will predominate and complexes of Fe^{+3} -ascorbate will tend to destabilize.

As the pH is raised several chemical events occur which tend to redirect the flow in Figure 6 which was just outlined. As pointed out previously, the hydrates of Fe^{+3} and Fe^{+2} begin to lose protons as the pH is raised, thus forming their respective hydroxides which are increasingly less soluble, with the standard reduction potential of $Fe(OH)_3$ (s) + e $\rightarrow$ Fe $(OH)_2$ (s) = $(OH)^-$ (aq) being -560mv. This means that at high pH values the standard reduction potentials of the two half reactions favor the formation of $Fe(OH)_3$ and reaction 1 (Figure 6) will go to the left, a condition opposite to that which occurs at low pH values.

Since most foods have a standard reduction potential of +400 mv or less, the formation of $Fe(OH)_3$ can occur with or without ascorbate. Therefore, the contribution of ascorbate as the pH is raised would seem to be to maintain the Fe^{+3} form in solution by forming a reasonably stable Fe^{+3} -ascorbate complex, thus favoring the downward direction of reaction 2 (Figure 6) and thereby promoting more oxidation to Fe^{+3} by indirectly favoring the leftward flow in equation 1 (Figure 6). Such stability was found by Conrad and Schade (44) at pH values from 4 to 9.

Thus, at high pH values, the overall effect which would be noted in a solution of iron and ascorbate would be oxidation.

This postulation for a reaction pathway to explain the seemingly contradictory data which implicates ascorbic acid as both a reductant and oxidant is not intended to be a final explanation. However, it does seem to fit many of the observations in the literature which under other explanations seem to be almost impossible from a chemical standpoint or simply to be contradictory.

Conrad and Schade (44) could not form a soluble Fe^{+3} -ascorbate complex starting at an alkaline pH, but could at an acid pH and found it to be stable even under alkaline conditions. This suggests that from a practical viewpoint, fortification might be best accomplished with an acid solution containing ascorbic acid and iron III or some purified extract of the ferric-ascorbate complex analagous to Saltman's suggestion for the use of a ferric fructose complex. However, Sayers et al (49) suggests that even if a feasible method were found for supplementing foods with ascorbic acid and inorganic iron, nutritional benefits would only be anticipated with uncooked or boiled foods since they found that ascorbic acid efficacy was lost due to oxidative destruction at the high temperatures required for baking.

In order to more fully understand the mode of action of ascorbic acid and substantiate the foregoing hypothesis, we are currently investigating the stability constants of the complexes in much more detail.

The thermodynamic stability constants between Fe^{+2} -ascorbate and Fe^{+3}- ascorbate are important since their relative values will not only affect the stability and amount of Fe^{+2} or Fe^{+3} in solution but also will affect the reaction flow as shown in Figure 6, and determine to some extent the exchange of iron with other ligands in food as well as with the biological transfer of iron to transferrin. However, Forth and Rummel (50) argue that the thermodynamic stability constants of iron are of limited value in defining the stability of complexes and chelates in biological media. They base this view on the observation that the thermodynamic stability constant is an equibilibrium constant determined in a definite medium and as such provides no information regarding the velocity of association and dissociation of complexes, especially when the complex formation takes place in the presence of competing ligands or metals and in association with oxidoreduction processes. In other words, they state, a high thermodynamic stability constant does not indicate that a complex is inert. Therefore, they propose that when assessing the stability of iron complexes in biological media, one is interested in the kinetic rather than the thermodynamic stability and they suggest that the half-time of the iron exchange of complexes can be used as a measure of the kinetic stability based in part on the extensive studies of Aaso _et al_ (51), Bates _et al_ (52, 53), and Billups _et al_ (54). It can be seen in Table IV that despite the small differences in the thermodynamic stability constants, these iron chelates have very different kinetic stabilities as measured by the exchange of iron with transferrin, a biological acceptor for iron.

This argument is logical and scientifically accurate with respect to the transfer of iron in the body. However, it does not address the potential importance of the thermodynamic stability constants of the two common valence forms of iron (II and III) with ligands in food.

When iron is added to a food the environment is going to affect the valence state as has been discussed previously. One of the parameters which might maintain a particular valence state in the face of adverse environmental conditions, such as pH or redox potential, is the stability of its complex. Therefore, either the Fe^{+2} or Fe^{+3} form might be maintained if one formed a complex with a greater thermodynamic stability than the other as discussed previously. Therefore, it would seem that the importance of the thermodynamic stability constant should not be discounted because it could have a great deal of relevance with respect to solubility and maintenance of a specific iron valence within a given food system.

Nojeim and Clydesdale (43) and Nojeim _et al_ (55) also attempted to utilize the results obtained in their model systems as a predictor of the effects of both pH and reduction potential of actual foods on the chemical status of iron. It would be most helpful to be able to predict the chemical fate of added iron simply by measuring the pH or reduction potential of the food.

Table IV. Kinetic stability of some Fe^{+3} chelates compared with their thermodynamic stability constants

Fe^{+3} Chelates of:	Thermodynamic Stability Constant	Half-Time of Iron Exchange with Iron-Free Transferrin (Kinetic Stability)
Nitrilotriacetic acid	23	3 sec.
Citric acid	25	8 hours
Ethylenediaminetetraacetic acid	25	4 days

In order to evaluate pH as a predictor of iron status in food, four iron sources, EI, FS, FOP and SFEDTA were added to three foods of different pH values; cranberry juice, tomato juice and a chemically leavened biscuit dough. The percent ionization and conversion to ferrous iron were measured and it was found that the chemical changes in the added iron followed the same trends observed in the phthalate buffers. Figures 7 and 8 show the results obtained with both the buffers and the foods in terms of the percentage ionization of the iron and the percentage of that ionized in the ferrous state, respectively. From these results, it may be seen that pH, though not quantitatively, is an important parameter to consider when predicting the general trends of chemical changes which iron might undergo when added to a food.

As pointed out previously the redox potential of the reduction of ferric to ferrous ion is +770 mv relative to the standard hydrogen electrode (SHE). This means that this reaction will be driven in the forward direction whenever ferric ion is present in a system whose overall redox potential is lower than +770 mv. How much lower the system is may be related to the level of completion to which the reaction is carried. Surprisingly, as pointed out by Nojeim (56), the study of reduction potentials as possible predictors of the chemical fate of iron in food has largely been neglected. In fact, literature discussing any effects of redox potential on food chemistry is sparse. Most of

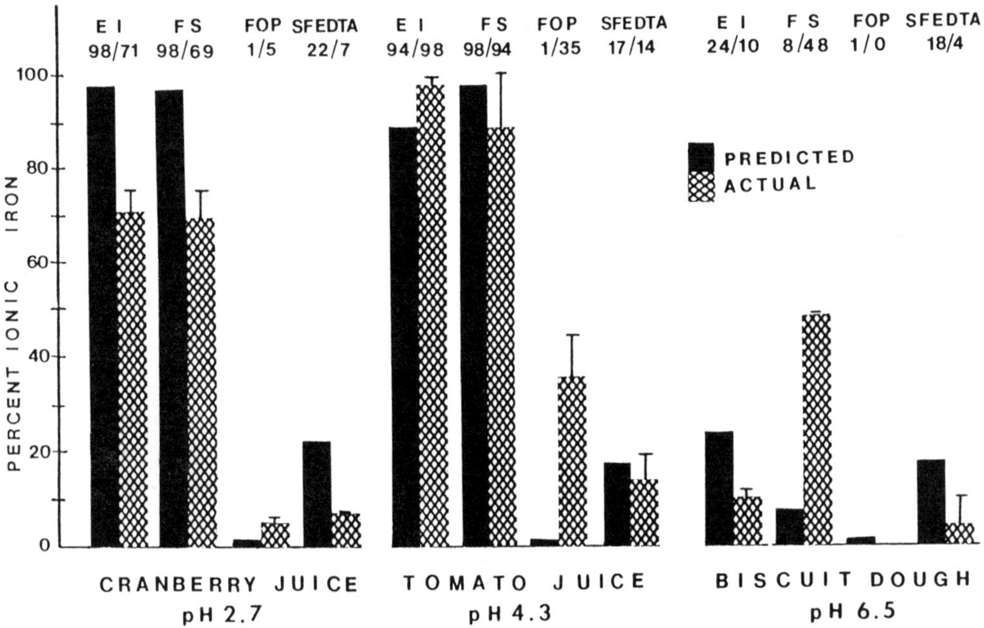

Figure 7. Percentage ionization of iron additives predicted by buffers and actually found in foods. EI, elemental iron; FS, ferrous sulfate; FOP, ferric orthophosphate; SFEDTA, sodium ferric EDTA trihydrate. (Reproduced, with permission, from Ref. 43. Copyright 1981, Institute of Food Technologists.)

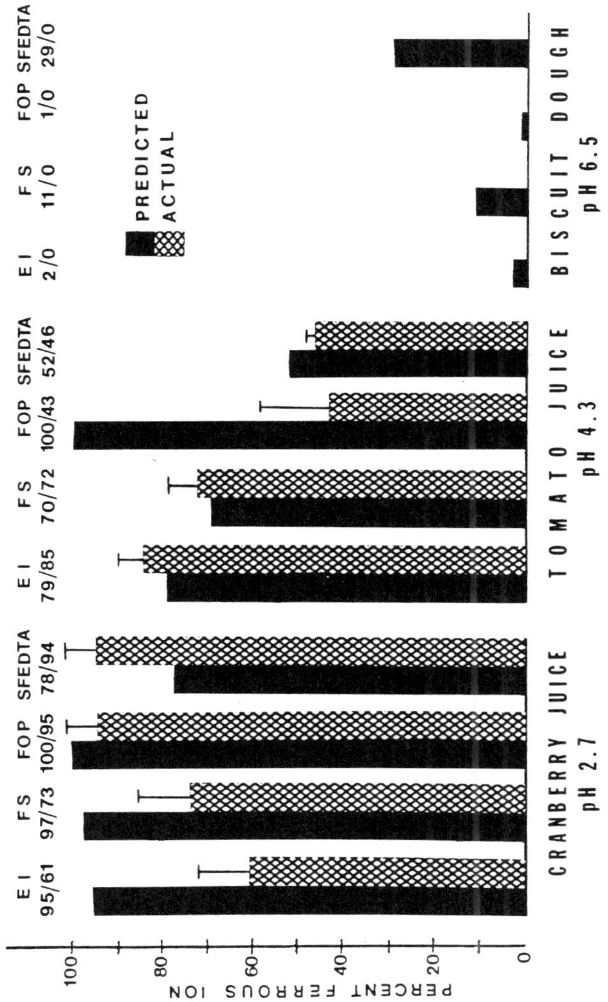

Figure 8. Percentage of ionized iron in the ferrous form predicted from buffers and actually found in foods. EI, elemental iron; FS, ferrous sulfate; FOP, ferric orthophosphate; SFEDTA, sodium ferric EDTA trihydrate. (Reproduced, with permission, from Ref. 43. Copyright 1981, Institute of Food Technologists.)

the work in this area has been on how redox potential affects microbial growth.

The first evidence of a relationship between redox potential and iron valence was observed by Kirch et al (57). A variety of iron fortified foods were subjected to an artificial gastric digestion with pepsin and/or HCl. After these treatments redox potential and pH measurements were recorded. Reduction of ferric to ferrous ion was also analyzed. It was found that pH and redox potential values were similar between each of the foods. This could have been a result of measurement after the acid/enzyme digestions. Redox potentials were all within 75 mv either way of +425 mv, SHE. Accordingly, reduction to ferrous ion was expected and observed. Where the degree of reduction was low, the degree of complex formation was high. In further work Bergeim and Kirch (58) studied the reduction of iron in actual gastric digestion. Samples were taken fron the stomachs of subjects shortly after ingestion of the same iron fortified foods studied previously. Results were comparable except that a greater degree of reduction of the iron in each food was observed *in vivo*. Even though no linear relationship was seen they concluded that the degree of reduction depends on the redox potential of the entire food system rather than on the concentration of one potent reducing compound present in a limited amount. In other words ascorbic acid added to an iron fortified food would not promote the reduction of ferric to ferrous ion unless the overall redox potential were favorable. This belief was supported through the research of Unnikrishnan et al (59) which involved the study of the effect of copper and microbial metabolism on oxidation-reduction reactions occurring in milk. These authors observed decreases in the redox potential of the system upon addition of reducing agents. The potential increased as ascorbic acid became oxidized to dehydroascorbic acid.

Reducing agents are often added to foods for their antioxidant properties. But even in foods devoid of these additives, there exist many innate redox couples. Endogenous electrochemically active compounds including vitamins C and E, organic acids, unsaturated fats, reducing sugars, quinones, oxygen and polyvalent metal ions all contribute to a food's overall redox potential. It should also be noted that these compounds and thus a food's redox potential are subject to changes during processing.

It seems apparent then, that the final form of iron in a food system should be directly influenced by the reduction potential of that system and anything which affects the reduction potential might affect the bioavailability of iron in the system. The enhancement of bioavailability of iron by the reducing compounds ascorbic acid and fructose is well known and has been discussed. However, it should be reemphasized that the addition of these, and other reducing agents, may in part increase iron bioavailability by their effect on redox potential as well as by their ability to form absorption enhancing chelates as suggested by Conrad and Schade (44) and Saltman (4).

Nojeim et al (55) utilized an electrolytic cell model system, free of oxygen, buffered with phthalate to pH 4.2 and designed to provide a redox potential between +300 and +650 mv to evaluate the effect of redox potential on the ionization and valence of four iron compounds; EI, FS, FOP, and SFEDTA, described previously (43). Data obtained were used to predict ionization and valence trends in actual food systems of different redox potentials. Redox potential was found to have no significant effect on the ionization of any of the four compounds evaluated. However, in the case of EI and FS lower potentials in the environment favored the reduced form of iron. This is to be expected since a greater difference between the +770 mv potential of the ferric to ferrous couple and the potential of its chemical environment would cause the reduction to be more spontaneous.

In the case of SFEDTA this trend seemed to be reversed and little effect was seen with FOP. This was probably due to the fact that in these two cases solubility was low (10%) producing a total of only 2.5 ppm in solution bringing into question the validity of the analytical technique used to differentiate the bivalent from the trivalent form.

In utilizing these results to predict ionization and valence in food materials; tomato juice (Eh=240), biscuit dough (Eh=340), cranberry juice (Eh=400) one would expect that the percentage iron ionized would be the same in each food since redox potential was found to have no effect in the model system on ionization. However research previously cited (43) showed that this was not the case as was seen in Figure 7. Obviously, this means that reduction potential of the food material is not a major factor in determining ionization of added iron.

Model system results were more consistent with actual foods, however, in the prediction of the amount of bivalent iron formed (Figure 9). The percentage ferrous iron was relatively high for all four iron compounds in tomato juice and cranberry juice where ionization was also high but not in biscuit dough where ionization was low.

This study shows a relationship, although not highly correlated, between redox and chemical behavior of iron, further emphasizing the need to evaluate reduction potentials prior to fortification.

The need to understand the chemical behavior of iron in foods is essential to a clear understanding of subsequent biological behavior. There are many factors which impinge upon the chemical status of iron in food with the physicochemical being only one. However, it is hoped that the interrelationship and importance of some of these factors might be considered more fully. In this way, a spirit of scientific cooperation might very well provide answers to the problems which seem to inhibit the existence of a population replete in terms of iron nutriture.

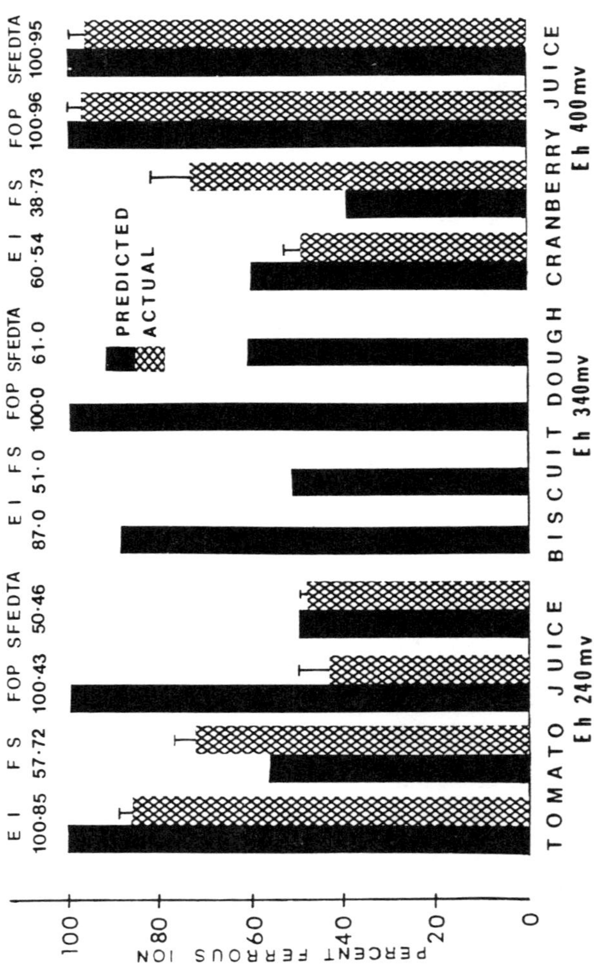

Figure 9. *Percentage of ionized iron in the ferrous state predicted from model systems with a known* Eh *and found in foods of varying* Eh *values. EI, elemental iron; FS, ferrous sulfate; FOP, ferric orthophosphate; SFEDTA, sodium ferric EDTA trihydrate. (Reproduced, with permission, from Ref. 55. Copyright 1981, Institute of Food Technologists.)*

Acknowledgments

This chapter is Paper No. 2050, Massachusetts Agricultural Experiment Station, University of Massachusetts at Amherst. This work was supported in part from Experiment Station Project No. NE-116 and a grant from the General Mills Foundation.

Literature Cited

1. U.S. Dept. of Agriculture, "Family Economics Review", Science & Education Administration, USDA, Beltsville, Md., Spring 1980, 22 pp.
2. Lee, K.; Clydesdale, F.M. CRC Critical Reviews in Food Science and Nutrition 1979, 11, 117.
3. Zoller, J.M.; Wolinsky, I.; Paden, C.A.; Hoskin, J.C.; Lewis, K.C.; Lineback, D.R.; McCarthy, R.D. Food Technol. 1980, 34, 38.
4. Saltman, P., J. Chem. Ed. 1965, 42, 682.
5. Spiro, T.G.; and Saltman, R. "Iron in Biochemistry and Medicine", Jacobs, A. and Wormwood, M. Eds. Academic Press, NY 1974.
6. Saltman, P.; Hegenauer, J.; Christopher, J. Ann. Clin. Lab Sci. 1976, 6, 167.
7. Pollack, S.; Kaufman, R.N.; Crosby, W.H. Blood 1964, 24. 577.
8. Bates, G.W.; Hegenauer, J.C.; Renner, J.; Saltman, P.; Spiro, G. Bioinorg. Chem 1973, 2, 311.
9. Heinrich, H.C.; Gabbe, E.E.; Bruggemann, J.; Oppitz, K.H. Nutr. Metab. 1974, 17, 236.
10. Loria, A.; Medal, L.S.; Elizando, J. Am. J. Clin. Nutr. 1962, 10, 124.
11. Rendleman, J.A. Jr. "Advances in Carbohydrate Chemistry"; Ed. Woltram, M. Academic Press, NY, 1966; 21, 209.
12. Amine, E.K.; Hegsted, D.M. J. Agric. Food Chem. 1975, 22, 470.
13. Derman, D.P.; Bothwell, T.H.; Torrance, J.D.; Bezwoda, W.R.; MacPhail, A.P.; Kew, M.C.; Sayers, M.H.; Disler, P.B.; Charlton, R.W. Br. J. Nutr. 43, 1980, 271.
14. Bachran, K.; Bernhard, R.A. J. Agric. Food Chem. 1980, 28, 536.
15. Layrisee, M.; Martinez-Torres, C. "Progress in Hematology", Vol. 7. Brown, E.B. and Moore, C.V. Eds. Grune and Stratton, NY, 1971; p 137.
16. Mahoney, A.W.; Hendricks, D.G. J. Food Sci. 1978, 43, 1473.
17. Van Campen, D. J. Nutr. 1973, 103, 139.
18. Welch, R.M.; Van Campen, D.R. J. Nutr. 1975, 105, 253.
19. Nelson, K.J.; Potter, N.N. J. Food Sci. 1979, 44, 104.
20. Nelson, K.J.; Potter, N.N. J. Food Sci. 1980, 45, 52.
21. Cheryan, M. CRC Critical Rev. Food Sci. Nutr. 1980, 13, 297.
22. Haug, A.; Smidsrod, O. Acta Chem. Schan. 1970, 24, 843.
23. Schweiger, R.G.; Kolloid-Z., Z. X. Polymere. 1966, 208, 28.
24. Camire, A.L.; Clydesdale, F.M. J. Food Sci. 1981, 46, 548.
25. Barry, J.A.; Halsey, G.D. Jr. J. Phys. Chem. 1963, 67, 1698.

26. Angyal, S.J. Pure Applied Chem. 1973, 35, 131.
27. Grant, G.T.; Morris, E.R.; Rees, D.A.; Smith, P.J.C.; Thorr,D. FEBS Letters 1973, 32, 195.
28. Furda, I. "Dietary Fibers, Chemistry and Nutrition", Ed. Inglett, G.E. and Falkehag, S.I. Academic Press: NY, 1979;p31.
29. Nagyvary, J.; Bradbury, E.L. Biochem and Biophysical Res. Comm. 1977, 77, 592.
30. Ranhotra, G.S.; Lee, C.; Gelroth, J.A.; Nutr. Rept. Intern. 1979, 19, 851.
31. Ranhotra, G.C.; Lee, C.; Gelroth, J.A.; Cereal Chem. 1979, 56, 156.
32. Lee, K.; Clydesdale, F.M. J. Food Sci. 1980, 45, 1500.
33. Anderson, N.E.; Clydesdale, F.M. J. Food Sci. 1980, 45, 1533.
34. Anderson, N.E.; Clydesdale, F.M. J. Food Sci. 1980, 45, 336.
35. Hodgkinson, A.; Zarembski, P.M. Calc. Tiss. Res. 1968, 2, 115.
36. Van Campen, D.R.; Welch, R.M. J. Nutr. 110, 1618.
37. Lynch, S.R., Cook, J.D. Ann. NY Acad. Sci. 1980, 355, 32.
38. Leichter, J.; Joslyn, M.A. Cereal Chem. 1967, 44, 346.
39. Lee, K.; Clydesdale, F.M. J. Food Sci. 1979, 44, 549.
40. Brise, H.; Hallberg, L. Acta. Med. Scand. Supp. 1962, (Stockholm) 171, (Supp. 376) 51.
41. Cook, J.D.; Monsen, E.R. Amer. J. Clin. Nutr. 1977, 30, 235.
42. Hodson, A.Z. J. Agric. Food Chem. 1980, 18, 946.
43. Nojeim, S.J.; Clydesdale, F.M.; J. Food Sci. 1981, 46, 606.
44. Conrad, M.E.; Schade, S.G. Gastroenterology. 1968, 55, 35.
45. Erdey, L.; Svehla, G. "Ascorbinometric Titrations". Akademiai Kiado, Budapest 1973; 183 pp.
46. Smith, G.J.; Dunkley, W.L. J. Dairy Sci. 1962, 45, 170.
47. Smith, G.J.; Dunkley, W.L. J. Food Sci. 1962, 27, 127.
48. Gorman, J.E.; Clydesdale, F.M. J. Food Sci. 1982, In press.
49. Sayers, M.H.; Lynch, S.R.; Jacobs, P.; Charlton, R.W.; Bothwell, T.W.; Walker, R.B.; Mayet, F. British J. Haem. 1973, 24, 209.
50. Forth, W.; Rummel, W. Physiol. Rev. 1973, 53, 724.
51. Aaso. R.; Malmström, B.G.; Saltman, R.; Vanngard, T. Biochem. Biophys. Acta. 1963, 75, 203.
52. Bates, G.W.; Billups, C.; Saltman, P. J. Biol. Chem. 1967, 242, 2810.
53. Bates, G.W.; Billups, C.; Saltman, P.; J. Biol. Chem. 1967, 242, 2816.
54. Billups, C.; Pape, L.; Saltman, P. J. Biol. Chem. 1967, 242, 4284.
55. Nojeim, S.J.; Clydesdale, F.M.; Zajicek, O.T. J. Food Sci. 1981, 46, 606.
56. Nojeim, S.J. "M.S. Thesis", Univ. of Mass., Amherst, MA 1981; 96 pp.
57. Kirch, E.R.; Bergeim, O.; Kleinberg, J.; James, J. J. Biol. Chem. 1947, 171, 687.
58. Bergeim, O.; Kirch, E.R. J. Biol. Chem. 1948, 172, 591.
59. Unnikrishnan, V.; Rao, D.S.; Rao, M.B. J. Milk and Food Tech. 1976, 39, 397.

RECEIVED June 2, 1982.

5

Ascorbic Acid: An Enhancing Factor in Iron Absorption

ELAINE R. MONSEN

University of Washington, Division of Human Nutrition, Dietetics, and Foods and Department of Medicine, Seattle, WA 98195

Ascorbic acid concomitantly consumed enhances nonheme iron absorption 3-6 fold: a key factor in the model estimating bioavailable dietary iron. The 500 mgs iron store Reference Individual is assumed to absorb 23% of ingested heme iron (estimated at 40% of meat, fish or poultry iron) and 3-8% of ingested nonheme iron (plant iron plus remaining meat, fish, poultry iron). The quantity of enhancing factors consumed at a specific meal, i.e. mgs ascorbic acid plus gms cooked meat/fish/poultry, determines % absorption of nonheme iron:

1. $\sum EF < 75$: $\% = 3 + 8.93 \log_n \left(\frac{EF + 100}{100}\right)$

2. $\sum EF \geq 75$: $\% = 8$

HANES 2 (1976 - 80) reports low intake of iron and ascorbic acid for large population segments, especially females below poverty line, e.g. at 10th percentile 4 mg iron and 7 mg ascorbic acid per day.

Prevention of iron deficiency in populations not sustaining chronic blood loss is possible by judicious selection of diets which enhance the bioavailability of dietary iron. The recent decades have produced significant research on the availability of iron as it is affected by various dietary components, those which enhance as well as those which inhibit iron absorption. This has allowed for the first time the quantification of dietary effects on a trace metal and the development of a model whereby the quantity of bioavailable iron in a diet may be estimated.

This paper will discuss four related areas: the major

0097-6156/82/0203-0085$06.00/0

section will be focused on the role of ascorbic acid in nonheme iron absorption; the second section will discuss briefly the model for estimating the quantity of available iron; the third section will deal with current estimates of dietary intake of iron and ascorbic acid in the United States; and the last section will discuss briefly the interrelationships of ascorbic acid and iron in abnormal states of metabolism.

The role of ascorbic acid in nonheme iron absorption

Radioisotope techniques have allowed precise measurement of dietary iron absorption. Initial studies utilized test meals of individual food which had been intrinsically labeled with radioactive iron prior to harvesting (1,2). Utilization of these single food meals allowed a rank order to be established among the tested foods. Subjects could serve as their own controls when an identical reference dose was given to each subject. This reference dose of ferrous sulfate:ascorbic acid was absorbed at a higher rate in iron deficient subjects than in iron replete subjects; a ratio of the absorption of the test meal to the reference dose allowed comparisons to be made between individual subjects. As these early studies were limited to study of single food items an effort was made to extend the technique by developing designs utilizing extrinsically tagged test meals (3,4). Utilization of these techniques has given evidence that dietary iron forms two separate pools in the gut, one a pool of heme iron and the other a pool of nonheme iron. The predominate source of iron in human diets is in the form of nonheme iron (5).

Ascorbic acid as an enhancing factor in nonheme iron absorption has been frequently observed. Callender, et al., fed intrinsically labeled hen eggs in a breakfast meal composed of bread, butter, jam, eggs, and tea or coffee to 26 subjects; when an addition of 100 mls of orange juice was added to this meal absorption increased to 280% of the control meal (6). Cook, et al., provided a meal of intrinsically labeled maize to subjects and observed that when 500 mgs of ascorbic acid was added that absorption of both intrinsic and extrinsically labeled iron was 6 times higher (3). Sayers, et al., utilized both intrinsically and extrinsically labeled maize, wheat and soybean, providing additional evidence of the applicability of the extrinsically labeled model (7). To the subjects whom they gave maize and 50 mgs of ascorbic acid, absorption was increased from 8.8% to 14.9%; to those subjects given maize plus 100 mg of ascorbic acid absorption was increased to 22.6%. The importance of the processing procedure was indicated in that the test meals to which ascorbic acid was added prior to high temperature baking, no enhancement of iron absorption was observed, suggesting that the high temperatures inactivated the ascorbic acid.

Bjorn-Rasmussen gave meals of maize plus 4.5 mgs of iron; to these meals were added 0-200 mgs of ascorbic acid (8). Incremental increases in iron absorption were observed as ascorbic acid was increased. In another study, Cook and Monsen gave 63 male subjects 700 kilocalorie meals composed of semi-synthetic ingredients of dextrimaltose, corn oil and ovalbumin; to these meals were added ascorbic acid ranging from 0 to 1000 mgs (9). With each increase in ascorbic acid an increase in iron absorption occurred. The rate of absorption appeared to be logarithmically related to the ascorbic acid content. It was further shown in this experiment that ascorbic acid must be present in the stomach at the same time that the nonheme iron is present. Nonheme iron was absorbed at a high rate from meals into which the ascorbic acid was incorporated. However if the ascorbic acid was given 4 or 8 hours before the test meal there was no enhancing effect observed.

Several investigators have looked at the effect of mixtures of foods on nonheme iron absorption. Layrisse tested meals that are reminiscent of those within various regional areas of Venezuela: nonheme iron was absorbed at a higher rate from meals that included ascorbic acid containing foods, the highest rate resulting from meals containing 66 mgs of ascorbate contributed by 150 gms of papaya (10). Hallberg, et al., tested 37 subjects with a diet consisting of a mixture of rice, cabbage, collards, string beans, chili paste, fish sauce and coconut cream (11). When a fruit mixture containing banana, papaya and oranges was added to this vegetal mixture, absorption was reported to increase three fold. Ascorbic acid content was calculated from food tables as being 35 mgs. Further addition of 80 gms of lean beef to the vegetal and fruit meal had an additive effect and enhanced the absorption of the basal diet six-fold.

Rossander, et al., tested the impact of adding 150 mls of orange juice to a breakfast consisting of bread, butter, marmalade, cheese and coffee; with the addition of the orange juice, absorption increased from 3.7% to 8% (12). When the breakfast meal included tea in place of coffee, the enhancing effect of the orange juice was less pronounced. A recent study compared vegetarian meals (13). The first composed of beans, rice, cornbread and apples contained 7 mg ascorbic acid: nonheme iron absorption was 2.2%; the second meal, composed of cauliflower, red kidney beans, white bread, cottage cheese and pineapple, contained 74 mg ascorbic acid: from this meal 16.9% of the nonheme iron was absorbed.

Reviewing the studies in which nonheme iron absorption has been assessed at various levels of ascorbic acid in test meals composed of either single food items or food mixtures it appears that, within any individual study, additional increments of ascorbic acid consistently increased absorption of nonheme iron (Table 1). Considering the wide differences in experimental conditions, the various studies incorporating 12.5 to 1000 mg ascorbic acid indicate clearly the enhancing effect that ascorbic acid has on nonheme iron absorption.

Table 1
The Effect of Ascorbic Acid on Absorption of Nonheme Iron in Humans

Ascorbic Acid mg.	Test Meal	Iron Absorption Ratio + Ascorbic Acid / - Ascorbic Acid	Ref.
12.5	Maize	1.3	8
25	700 Kcal SS*	1.7	9
25	Maize	3.0	8
35	Vegetal meal ± fruits	2.7	11
50	Maize	1.7	7
50	700 Kcal SS	2.5	9
50	Maize	2.6	8
50	Bread, egg, ± orange juice	2.8	6
66	Maize ± 150 g papaya	5.0	10
70	Bread, cheese, tea ± orange juice	1.2	12
70	Bread, cheese, coffee ± orange juice	2.2	12
74	600-700 Kcal vegetarian	7.7	13
100	Maize	2.6	7
100	700 Kcal SS	4.1	9
100	Maize	4.6	8
200	Maize	6.1	8
250	700 Kcal SS	4.7	9
500	Maize	6.0	3
500	700 Kcal SS	6.2	9
1000	700 Kcal SS	9.6	9

*Semi-synthetic meal composed of dextrimaltose, corn oil and ovalbumin.

Several dietary factors have been identified which inhibit nonheme iron absorption. Tea and tannates appear particularly inhibiting (14). Rossander, et al., reported only a slight increase in absorption when orange juice was added to a tea-containing breakfast meal (12). Other food additives such as EDTA may have an inhibiting effect on nonheme iron absorption if the EDTA is in high molar concentrations relative to nonheme iron (15).

Ascorbic acid has also been shown to interact with therapeutic iron. Derman, et al., have reported that ascorbic acid increases absorption of various iron fortification compounds in infant formulas in cereals; this three-fold increase in iron absorption induced by ascorbic acid was observed in multiparous women (16). El-Hawary, et al., studied 97 infants and young children and observed that ascorbic acid increased absorption from a four mg iron supplement as ferrous sulfate (17). McPhail, et al., have also reported increases in absorption of iron from either ferrous sulfate or iron:EDTA with incorporation of three to six molar concentrations of ascorbic acid (18). When these mixtures of ascorbic acid and iron fortification compounds were added to foods such as maize porridge before the foods were cooked absorption was not enhanced.

Estimating bioavailable iron in the diet

Extensive research on the absorption of iron from various types of meals has allowed guidelines to be developed by which the amount of dietary iron available for absorption may be estimated. Iron is the first trace mineral to be thus treated and thus serves as a model for other nutrients (19). The model for estimating bioavailable iron is based on the concept that iron forms a) a pool of heme iron which is readily available to humans and is uneffected by other dietary components and b) a pool of nonheme iron which is of low bioavailability unless enhancing factors are present concommitantly (20).

Recognition is made of the importance of the extent of an individual's iron stores as it will influence the amount of nonheme iron and heme iron that would be absorbed. The conservative model suggests utilization of an individual with 500 mgs of iron stores as the reference individual for whom bioavailable iron may be calculated. As the purpose of such a model is to compare one diet with another, it is immaterial what level of iron stores an individual has in that the comparison between diets will not be affected. The calculated values will, of course, be lower for the amount of total available iron with an individual with moderate iron stores of 500 mgs than they would be for an individual with zero iron stores.

The enhancing factors considered for the absorption of nonheme iron are ascorbic acid and meat, fish and poultry. The earlier model classified meals as low, moderate or high availability; this produced artificial stair step increments. Thus, the model has been further refined to show that the enhancing factors are additive in their effect and smoothly increase dietary nonheme iron absorption in a logarithmic fashion (21). Thus the amount of nonheme iron available for absorption from each meal or snack can be estimated from the summation of enhancing factors (milligrams of ascorbic acid plus grams of cooked meat/fish/poultry). Absorption of nonheme iron for the reference individual with 500 mg iron stores is assumed to change from 3% for a meal with no enhancing factors to 8% from a meal of 75 enhancing factors. The formulas for calculating the rate of absorption of nonheme iron for the reference individual are:

$$\text{For EF} < 75: \quad \%\ \text{bioavailability of nonheme iron} = 3 + 8.93 \log_n\left(\frac{EF + 100}{100}\right)$$

$$\text{For EF} \geq 75: \quad \%\ \text{bioavailability of nonheme iron} = 8$$

Absorption of heme iron is estimated to be 23% for the reference individual. Heme iron may be estimated at 40% of the iron in meat, fish and poultry. Nonheme iron would be calculated as the remaining 60% of meat, fish and poultry iron plus the iron in vegetables, grain and other foods. The available nonheme iron and heme iron from each meal and snack can be summed to calculate the total day's available iron.

Dietary intake of iron and ascorbic acid

Preliminary data (22) from the second Health and Nutrition Examination Survey, 1976–1980 (HANES 2) indicates a mean intake of iron for females at 10.6 mgs per day (Table 2A). This level is 10% higher than HANES 1. A higher nutrient density exhibited by milligrams of iron per thousand kilocalories was seen in each age group, although the mean intake of iron is below the Recommended Dietary Allowances (19) for females during their reproductive and menstruating years. The males also show a higher iron intake and higher nutrient density in HANES 2 compared to HANES 1 (Table 2B). Ascorbic acid intake (Tables 3A & B) report the mean intake of ascorbic acid to be above the Recommended Dietary Allowances in all age groups.

Considering the intake data at various percentile levels, new interpretations come forward. In all cases the values are skewed toward the upper intake levels, thus all subjects at the 50th percentile report consumption below the mean intake level. For women at the 25th percentile the average intake was approximately 7 mg of iron per day and at the 10th percentile the intake was down to only 5 mg per day. The males at the 25th

Table 2A
IRON INTAKE (mg)
FEMALES
HANES 2, 1976-1980

	All Income Levels				Income Below Poverty		
Percentile:	Mean	50th	25th	10th	50th	25th	10th
6 mon-74 yrs	10.6	9.6	6.9	5.0	8.8	6.3	4.3
6-11 mon	12.9	9.4	4.8	3.4	7.8	3.5	2.3
1-2 yrs	8.5	7.0	5.1	3.6	7.1	5.0	3.4
3-5	9.5	8.5	6.4	4.6	9.0	6.4	4.4
6-8	10.8	10.1	7.8	5.9	9.8	7.6	5.5
9-11	11.4	10.2	7.5	5.8	9.6	5.9	5.7
12-14	10.8	9.9	6.8	5.3	8.5	5.5	4.7
15-17	9.9	9.4	6.3	4.4	9.8	6.8	5.0
18-24	10.6	9.7	6.8	4.6	8.8	6.1	3.8
25-34	10.9	9.7	7.0	4.9	10.3	6.4	4.5
35-44	11.2	10.0	7.5	5.3	8.6	6.0	4.2
45-54	10.4	9.5	7.3	5.5	8.4	6.0	4.5
55-64	10.7	9.4	7.0	5.2	7.8	5.5	4.0
64-74	10.2	9.0	6.6	5.1	8.0	6.0	4.3

Table 2B
IRON INTAKE (mg)
MALES
HANES 2, 1976-1980

	All Income Levels				Income Below Poverty		
Percentile:	Mean	50th	25th	10th	50th	25th	10th
6 mon-74 yrs	15.5	13.8	9.7	7.0	12.2	8.2	5.7
6-11 mon	12.8	8.2	4.3	2.6	8.3	4.2	2.2
1-2 yrs	8.7	7.4	5.2	3.6	7.3	4.9	3.4
3-5	10.5	9.2	7.0	5.2	9.5	7.0	5.1
6-8	12.5	11.4	8.8	6.6	11.4	8.7	5.7
9-11	14.4	13.1	9.1	7.2	11.7	7.6	6.3
12-14	15.9	14.4	9.9	7.5	11.7	8.1	6.3
15-17	17.4	15.0	10.6	7.2	14.3	10.2	6.6
18-24	17.8	15.7	10.9	7.7	15.8	10.4	6.6
25-34	17.3	15.6	11.2	8.0	15.2	10.0	6.4
35-44	16.0	14.6	10.8	7.9	11.9	7.9	5.3
45-54	16.2	14.5	11.2	8.1	15.4	11.1	8.4
55-64	14.8	13.4	10.1	7.3	11.1	8.1	5.3
65-74	14.1	12.3	9.1	6.7	10.4	7.4	4.8

Table 3A
ASCORBIC ACID INTAKE (mg)
FEMALES
HANES 2, 1976-1982

	All Income Levels				Income Below Poverty		
Percentile:	Mean	50th	25th	10th	50th	25th	10th
6 mon-74 yrs	93	63	27	11	44	19	7
6-11 mon.	72	51	31	13	51	34	21
1-2 yrs.	86	64	27	13	61	23	12
3-5	96	68	29	15	54	24	10
6-8	109	80	34	19	80	36	18
9-11	94	59	32	17	43	19	13
12-14	83	56	25	11	33	16	3
15-17	73	42	21	9	31	14	3
18-24	92	59	25	9	46	20	6
25-34	92	55	24	9	36	19	7
35-44	83	53	23	10	32	13	4
45-54	97	69	26	9	62	15	4
55-64	107	88	35	15	47	20	7
65-74	105	90	37	13	71	24	8

Table 3B
ASCORBIC ACID INTAKE (mg)
MALES
HANES 2, 1976-1980

	All Income Levels				Income Below Poverty		
Percentile:	Mean	50th	25th	10th	50th	25th	10th
6 mon-74 yrs	108	73	33	15	57	23	9
6-11 mon.	63	51	23	14	41	19	12
1-2 yrs.	90	64	28	13	46	20	9
3-5	104	76	34	16	72	33	12
6-8	105	68	34	19	52	26	15
9-11	119	88	41	20	76	37	15
12-14	123	72	32	15	51	22	12
15-17	112	69	33	16	55	23	10
18-24	129	76	35	14	72	36	12
25-34	108	66	31	13	48	18	5
35-44	96	66	28	15	46	17	3
45-54	102	76	34	13	80	24	7
55-64	103	82	34	15	52	23	6
65-74	100	79	33	11	45	11	3

percentiles remain around 10 mg per day and at the 10th percentile are approximately 8 mg of iron per day. Ascorbic acid intakes at the 25th percentile for the females are under 30 mg per day and at the 10th percentile they average only 11 mg per day. Males are slightly higher, being 33 and 15 mg per day respectively at the 25th and 10th percentile.

Individuals whose incomes are below poverty line have even lower intakes of iron and of ascorbic acid. At these low income levels the females at the 50th percentile report daily intakes of only 9 mg of iron; this drops to 6 mg at the 25th percentile and to only 4 mg iron per day at the 10th percentile. This level of intake is only 22% of the Recommended Dietary Allowance for the menstruating woman. The intake of the males whose income is below poverty line is reduced to 6 mg of iron per day at the 10th percentile. Ascorbic acid is also dramatically reduced in intake for those individuals below the poverty line. At the 25th percentile the females below poverty consume on an average under 20 mg of ascorbic acid a day and at the 10th percentile their average intake is only 7 mg per day. The males faired slightly better, being slightly above 20 mg at the 25th percentile and around 9 mg of ascorbic acid per day at the 10th percentile. Groups at and below the 25th percentile, particularly those below the poverty line, are vulnerable to dietary iron deficiency due to low dietary intake of iron; plus it is highly likely that these same people have low ascorbic acid intakes and thus the limited amount of dietary iron they consume is apt to be poorly absorbed. Although on average the US intake appears to be sufficient for ascorbic acid and certainly for iron in the male, the intake of these nutrients appears to be dangerously low for a substantial portion of the population.

A study has recently been completed which indirectly indicates that high dietary quality can provide the nutrients necessary for iron absorption utilization. This was a study done in a 176 high frequency blood donors who were able to maintain hemoglobin levels considered adequate to donate blood over an extended period of time (23). These blood superdonors donated 17 units of blood over a four year period. Although their iron stores were very low, these subjects were maintaining hemoglobin and hematocrit levels above standard minimum levels. These volunteers were queried as to their dietary intakes; their diets were of unusually high quality with regard to both ascorbic acid intake and meat, fish and poultry.

Ascorbic acid:Iron and relationships in abnormal state of metabolism

Ascorbic acid and iron interrelate in a variety of conditions where iron stores are either greatly reduced or dramatically increased. In untreated idopathic hemochromatosis (Brissot, et al., 1978), white blood cell ascorbic acid is dramatically reduced; it is assumed that this decrease in ascorbic acid status results from iron overload (24). Chatterjea, et al., has reported that platelet ascorbic acid is particularly low in thalassemia, while it is higher than normal in iron deficiency anemia (25). Giving iron salts as the therapy for iron deficiency anemia reduced the ascorbic acid content in both platelets and leucocytes. Indeed reduced ascorbic acid stores have been shown to be beneficial to individuals with thalassemia major when the thalassemia was treated with blood transfusions and iatrogenic iron overload produced; a scorbutic condition developed despite adequate intake of vitamin C with this high iron overload. The vitamin C deficiency however appeared to protect the tissues from damage due to the iron overload. When chelation therapy is utilized, ascorbic acid status needs to be monitored very carefully (26).

Extensive research has been conducted in guinea pigs whereby relationships between ascorbic acid and iron were studied. Alterations in spleen and hepatic iron levels of hemosiderin and ferritin as well as changes in hepatic microsomal cytochrome P-450 have been observed with ascorbic acid deficiency (27-29).

Ascorbic acid as panacea for iron deficiency

The importance of iron in nutritional status has been recognized for centuries. In an effort to dissolve iron and make it more available numerous therapies have been devised including such rarities as syrups of sherry in which iron wire has been soaked for 30 days, slices of apple into which iron nails have been imbedded, and solutions of vinegar into which iron filings have been placed weeks earlier. The interaction of ascorbic acid and iron has been recognized more recently (30). It may be that the most useful and readily found therapy for iron deficiency will be dietary ascorbic acid which has the capability of increasing the rate of nonheme iron absorption several fold.

Literature Cited

1. Moore, C.V.; Dubach, R. Trans. Assoc. Am. Physicians 1951, 64, 245-256.
2. Layrisse, M.; Cook, J.D.; Martinez, C.; Roche, M.; Kuhn, I. N.; Walker, R.B.; Finch, C.A. Blood 1969, 33: 430-443.
3. Cook, J.D.; Layrisse, M.; Martinez-Torres, C.; Walker, R.; Monsen, E.R.; Finch, C.A. J. Clin. Invest. 1972; 51:801-815.
4. Heinrich, H.C.; Bartels, H.; Gabbe, E.E.; Kugler, G.; Oppitz, K.H. Arzneim. Forsch. (Drug Res.). 1972, 22:1091-1103.
5. Bull, N.L.; Buss, D.H. J Human Nutr 1980, 34:141-5.
6. Callender, S.T.; Marney, S.R.; Warner, G.T. Brit. J. Haematol. 1970, 19:657-665.
7. Sayers, M.H.; Lynch, S.R.; Jacobs, P.; Charlton, R.W.; Bothwell, T.H.; Walker, R.B.; Mayet, F. Brit. J. Haematol. 1973, 24:209-218.

8. Bjorn-Rasmussen, E.; Hallberg, L. Nutr. Metabol. 1974, 16: 94-100.
9. Cook, J.D.; Monsen, E.R. Am.J.Clin.Nutr. 1977, 30:235-241.
10. Layrisse, M.; Martinez-Torres, C.; Gonzalez, M. Am. J. Clin.Nutr. 1974, 27:152-162.
11. Hallberg, L.; Garby, L.; Suwanik, R.; Bjorn-Rasmussen, E. Am. J. Clin.Nutr. 1974, 27:826-836.
12. Rossander, L.; Hallberg, L.; Bjorn-Rasmussen, E. Am. J. Clin. Nutr. 1979, 32:2484-2489.
13. Hallberg, L. Am. J. Clin. Nutr. 1981, 34:2242-2247.
14. Disler, P.B.; Lynch, S.R.; Charlton, R.W.; Torrance, J.D.; Bothwell, T.H.; Walker, R.B.; Mayet, F. Gut 1975, 16:193-200.
15. Cook, J.D.; Monsen, E.R. Am. J. Clin. Nutr. 1976, 29:614-620.
16. Derman, D.P.; Bothwell, T.H.; MacPhail, A.P.; Torrance, J.D.; Bezwoda, W.R.; Charlton, R.W.; Mayet, F.G.H. Scand. J. Haematol. 1980, 25:193-201.
17. El-Hawary, M.F.S.; El-Shobaki, F.A.; Kholeif, T. Br. J. Nutr. 1975, 33:351-355.
18. MacPhail, A.P.M.; Bothwell, T.H.; Torrance, J.D.; Derman, D.P.; Bezwoda, W.R.; Charlton, R.W. Br. J. Nutr. 1981, 45 215-227.
19. National Research Council, Food and Nutrition Board. "Recommended Dietary Allowances, 9th Ed." National Academy of Sciences, Washington, DC, 1980.
20. Monsen, E.R.; Hallberg, L.; Layrisse, M.; Hegsted, D.M.; Cook, J.D.; Mertz, W.; Finch, C.A. Am. J. Clin. Nutr. 1978, 31:134-141.
21. Monsen, E.R.; Balintfy, J.L. J. Am. Dietet. Assoc. 1982, 80: (4)307-311.
22. National Center for Health Statistics: Caloric and selected values for persons 6 months - 74 years of age, second Health and Nutrition Examination Survey, United States, 1976-1980. in preparation.
23. Monsen, E.R.; Donahue, D.; Critchlow, C.W.; Finch, C.A. Fed. Proc. 1982, 41:275.
24. Brissot, P.; Deugnier, Y.; LeTreut, A.; Regnouard, F.; Simon, M.; Bourel, M. Digestion 1978, 17:479-487.
25. Chatterjea, B.; Maitra, A.; Banerjee, D.K.; Basu, A.K. Acta haemat. 1980, 64:271-275.
26. Cohen, A.; Cohen, I.J.; Schwartz, E. New Engl. J. Med. 1981, 304:(3)158:160.
27. Smith, C.H.; Bidlack, W.R. Biochem. Med. 1980; 24:43-48.
28. Milne, D.B.; Omaye, S.T. Internat J. Vit. Res. 1980, 50: 301-308.
29. Roeser, H.P.; Halliday, J.W.; Sizemore, D.J.; Nikles, A.; Willgoss, D. Brit. J. Haemat. 1980, 45:457-466.
30. Lynch, S.R.; Cook, J.D. Ann. N.Y. Acad. Sci. 1980 355 32-44.

RECEIVED August 5, 1982.

6

Influence of Copper, Zinc, and Protein on Biological Response to Dietary Iron

W. O. CASTER and ANNA V. A. RESURRECCION[1]

University of Georgia, Home Economics, Foods, and Nutrition, Athens, GA 30602

Rat diets containing iron concentrations differing over a 300-fold range were fed for 30 days. Different diets also contained 8.5-20% protein (casein and/or mixed-grain protein) with or without supplements of copper and/or zinc. Zinc had no effect, but copper and protein had major effects as observed by measuring hemoglobin, hematocrit, red cell counts and liver iron. Most profound anemia was seen with 20% protein and low intakes of iron and copper.

Some time ago Caster and Parthemos (1) fed common breakfast cereals to groups of young rats and noted the biochemical and physiological changes that occurred within the next month as a result of that diet. Among changes observed were a number (2) that were not easily anticipated on the basis of the known nutrient intake information. Of significance to the present discussion was the observation that there were substantial differences in hemoglobin concentration and in the amount of iron stored in the liver. As Figure 1 shows, there was an inverse relationship between these two sets of data.

Some diets, including the oatmeal diet (shown as a circle) produced rats with high hemoglobin concentrations but with minimal amounts of iron stored in the liver. At the other extreme (shown as squares) were some of the most widely advertised ready-to-eat cereals made from a mixture of grains enriched with all vitamins and minerals (including iron) for which human requirements have been established. These yielded animals with lower hemoglobin levels but with large amounts of iron stored in the liver. Over the entire series of diets tested (3) there was a negative correlation ($P < 0.01$) between the hemoglobin concentration and the amount of iron stored in the liver.

[1] Current address: Pennsylvania State University, Department of Food Science, University Park, PA 16802

0097-6156/82/0203-0097$06.00/0

This observation seems to run directly counter to common assumptions (4) that, over the normal range of hemoglobin levels, the concentration of hemoglobin in the blood is directly related to the body iron stores (and to the amount and nutritional availability of iron in the diet). As such, this situation seemed worthy of further experimental study.

In response to this, experimental work was carried out in two directions. Some work (5) involved studies with purified diets of known compositions. The other series of studies (6, 7) involved the addition of nutrient supplements to cereal diets (similar to those shown in Figure 1 as squares) to see if the observed biochemical effects could be reversed by adding selected nutrient supplements to the diet. It was in this latter supplementation work that it soon became evident that protein, copper and possibly zinc were nutrients of prime importance.

Experimental

In each experiment, groups of 6-12 male white rats were fed diets of controlled composition for 28-30 days. All rats were individually caged in a room with controlled temperature (25 ± 1°C) and a controlled light-dark cycle.

Control groups were fed commercial chow (Purina) or a complete diet prepared of purified components (8). The mineral mixture in this latter diet could be prepared without iron, copper or zinc so that these mineral elements could be added in controlled amounts as supplements in the form of ferrous sulfate, copper sulfate, or zinc carbonate. Under ether anesthesia, blood was removed from the abdominal aorta with a 1.5 inch, 22 gauge needle attached to a 10 ml syringe containing dried heparin. Aliquots were taken for hemoglobin, hematocrit, red cell counts and plasma analysis. The liver was removed, weighed, frozen and saved for analysis.

Hemoglobin was determined by the absorbance at 540 nm of a 1:200 dilution of blood with 0.4% ammonium hydroxide. An electronic counter (Coulter) was used to determine the red cell counts. In different parts of this work, the liver iron was determined spectrographically, with the ferrozine method (9) or with the use of 2,4,6-tripyridyl-1,3,5-triazine (10). Further experimental details, including identity of cereals involved, can be found in the initial reports (1, 3, 5, 6, 7).

Results

Figures 2-4 each contain two sets of data. One series of results (represented by circles) was obtained with rats consuming a diet containing 10% casein. The other (represented by triangles) was with diets containing 20% casein.

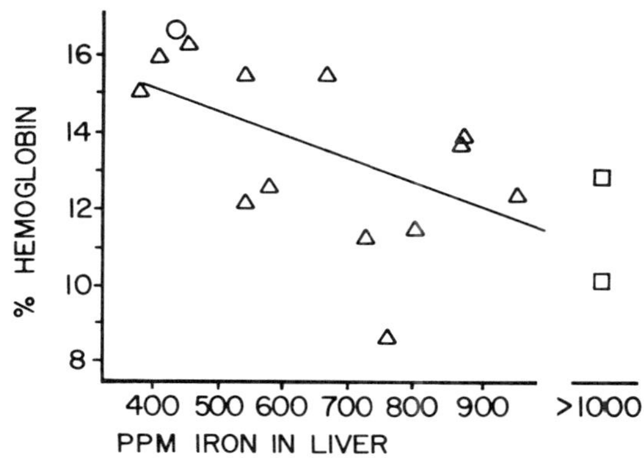

Figure 1. Relationship between the hemoglobin concentration in blood and the iron concentration in liver in rats fed different commercial breakfast cereals or control diets (3).

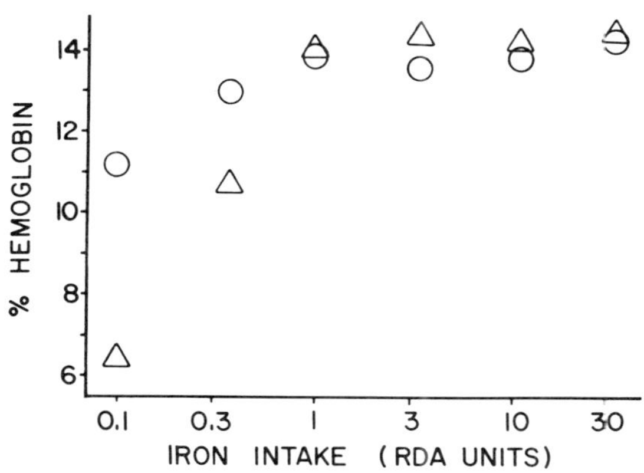

Figure 2. Effect of iron intake on the hemoglobin concentration in the rat. Diets contained either 10% (○) or 20% (△) protein (5).

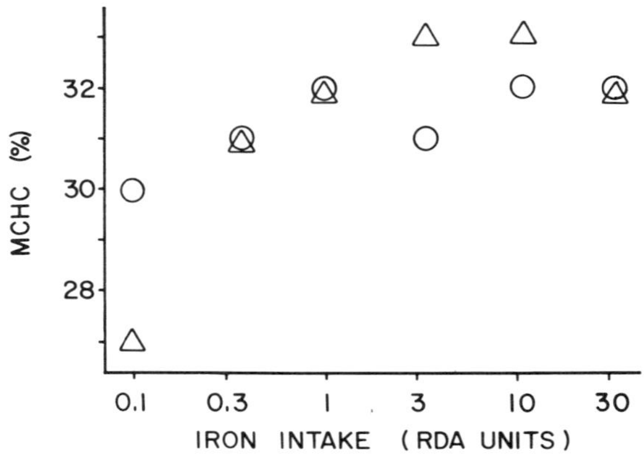

Figure 3. Effect of iron intake on the mean corpuscular hemoglobin concentration (MCHC) in the rat. Diets contained either 10% (○) or 20% (△) protein (5).

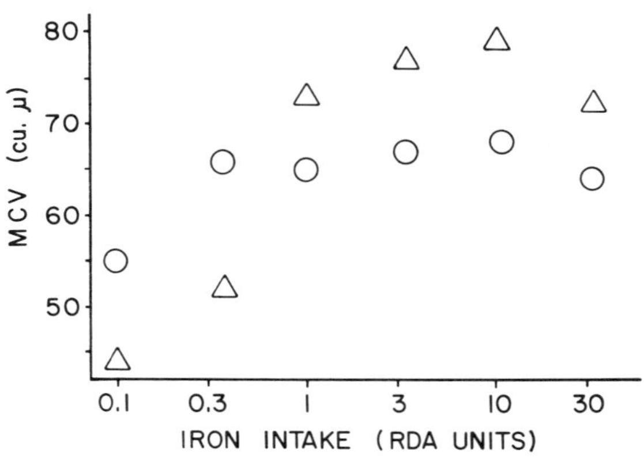

Figure 4. Effect of iron intake on the mean corpuscular volume (MCV) of the rat red cell. Diets contained either 10% (○) or 20% (△) protein (5).

When the rat is used as an experimental model in the study of problems important to human nutrition, there is always a question relative to the appropriate amount and type of protein to use in the rat diet. Casein is one of the few high quality proteins that is readily available in a reasonably pure and stable form. A committee of the American Institute of Nutrition suggests (11) that rat diets contain 20% casein. Those using rats in studies related to uremia and kidney failure (12) find excellent survival and performance with diets containing about 8% casein. The human Recommended Daily Allowance (RDA) for protein, during most of the growth years, is in the range of 6-10% of calories (13, 14). In malnourished and anemic human populations, the quantity and quality of protein in the diet might well be on the low side of this range. Historic evidence suggests that rats are quite capable of thriving on grains, human garbage, and other foods containing protein limited in both amount and quality. On this basis, it seemed reasonable to use diets containing 10% and 20% casein so as to obtain experimental results representative of a broad portion of this nutritionally interesting range.

In Figures 2-4 the iron intake values are expressed in RDA units and are plotted on a logarithmic scale so as to show response values over a wide range of intake levels.

Dose-Response Data Related to Dietary Iron. At the outset it seemed important to determine the nature of the dose-response curve relating dietary iron to blood hemoglobin levels.

On the basis of the data obtained with 20% protein diets (triangles in Figure 2), it is evident that the hemoglobin values are in good agreement with the generally recognized RDA for the rat (15). Above 35 ppm (one RDA unit) of iron in the diet, the hemoglobin values are substantially constant, and below this dietary intake the hemoglobin values drop off very rapidly and result in a serious anemia by the time one gets to 0.1 of the RDA.

Shown in Figure 2, however, there is another set of values--those represented by the open circles. These values were obtained from diets having 10% protein, and they show quite a different response pattern. It was anticipated that the low protein diet would make the iron-deficiency anemia more severe. This was not the case however. With 10% casein, one could proceed down to 0.3 RDA for iron (10 ppm) without any significant decrease in the hemoglobin level, and at 0.1 RDA (3 ppm iron) the hemoglobin level (though significantly lower) was not outside the range frequently seen in work with "normal" humans.

Both the hematocrit values and the red cell counts (5) show much the same story. When these values were used to compute the mean corpuscular hemoglobin concentration (Figure 3) and the mean cell volumes (Figure 4) it was found that indeed a microcytic hypochromic anemia had been produced at the lowest iron intake levels. However, the effect was much more pronounced when 20% protein was fed than when the diet contained 10% casein.

From these observations it is evident that the dose-response relationship between dietary iron and blood hemoglobin level is highly dependent upon the amount of protein in the diet. And indeed the different conclusions that have been expressed in relation to the iron requirement are only interpretable if one specifies the nature and amount of protein in the diet. One could extend this further and say that conclusions based on animal work, using high protein diets, may be of questionable value when one is interested in human experience with malnourished populations consuming diets with small amounts of low quality protein.

Supplementation of Cereals. The next chapter of the story comes from experience in supplementing these breakfast cereal diets with other nutrients. Initially, the breakfast cereal was supplemented in a factorial fashion with protein, a vitamin mixture and several mineral mixtures. Only protein and a trace mineral group containing copper and zinc showed significant effects (6). Next, individual nutrients and pairs of nutrients were tried (7).

In Table I it is seen that the addition of more iron was of no assistance in increasing the hemoglobin level. In this instance it actually decreased the hemoglobin and hematocrit levels slightly. Likewise, the concentration of iron in the liver was, if anything, increased. It was only when copper was added that one saw a measurable increase in hemoglobin and hematocrit levels. When both iron and copper were added, the effect was no better than when copper by itself was added. In this instance the diet contained 8.5% protein. This amount is basically what was present in the breakfast cereal without any further protein supplementation. Others have been quick to point out that this situation is not realistic because these cereals are typically consumed with milk. It is reasonable, therefore, to parallel this experiment with one in which casein is added to the diet.

Table II shows some of the results (7) obtained when the total protein was increased to 20%. A more severe anemia was observed. The addition of copper was, again, effective. If anything, it was even more effective than in the case of the low protein diet. Copper increased the hemoglobin level. It increased the hematocrit and even decreased the liver iron somewhat. This result was unexpected because, by direct analysis, the cereal already contained about half of the RDA for copper--and one would hardly anticipate that a small amount of added copper could have much effect under these conditions.

Discussion

The data seem to suggest that one of the significant nutrient deficiencies observed in the cereals shown as squares in Figure 1 related to copper. Both copper and protein are very important in determining the biological effects that one can expect to find with a given dose of iron. It appears that most of the effects

Table I. Effect of Supplementing the Basal Diet (8.5% mixed-grain protein) with Iron or Copper, or both Iron and Copper. Reprinted by permission from a larger table in the Science of the Total Environment (7).

	Basal	+Fe	+Cu	Fe+Cu
Hemoglobin (%)	10.4	9.2	11.3	9.8
Hematocrit (%)	31	28	38	30
Liver Fe (ppm)	183	198	187	211

Table II. Effect of Supplementing a High-Protein Diet (Basal plus 11.5% casein) with Iron or Copper, or both Iron and Copper. Reprinted by permission from a larger table in the Science of the Total Environment (7).

	Basal	+Fe	+Cu	+Fe+Cu
Hemoglobin (%)	7.4	8.2	12.7	13.4
Hematocrit (%)	24	25	39	42
Liver Fe (ppm)	138	133	96	123

observed in Figure 1 can be explained in terms of a deficiency of copper and the lack of high quality protein--perhaps coupled with an excess of iron.

In other parts of the work it was evident that the amount of protein, and possibly the type of protein, was crucial in determining the physiological response to a measured dose of iron. Zinc was present in some nutrient mixtures that were effective (6), and Klevay (16) has suggested that the zinc/copper interaction is an important determinant of plasma cholesterol concentration. We (17) failed to confirm this latter observation, and all trials with zinc as an independent variable provided negative results.

In view of the strong interactions with copper and protein it may be worth taking another look at the general concept of "the bioavailability of iron." For years we have considered that there is a net absorption of only about 10% of the dietary iron. Phytate and perhaps other factors tend to decrease this percentage. On the other hand, vitamin C and certain amino acids may increase the percentage of iron absorbed. It was in this context that one spoke of the various dietary factors as modifying the bioavailabilty of iron.

In general, if the bioavailability was low, the simple answer was to feed more iron. On this basis, the human RDA for iron has been increased to very high levels. In fact, the latest NRC report (14) carries "Footnote h" that indicates there is no way that the pregnant female can get enough iron from a practical diet. Iron supplementation is a necessity.

In the case shown in Figure 1, there was no real question about an inadequate amount of iron in the diet or an inadequate absorption of iron. In fact there was about a three-fold excess of iron in the crucial diets. The observed hemoglobin levels may have been low enough for some (4) to express clinical concern, but there was an excess of iron in the liver. The addition of more iron to the diet did not increase the hemoglobin. If anything, it decreased it. The major effect of feeding more iron was to increase the amount of iron stored in the liver.

It is clear that more than one metabolic process is subsumed under the term "bioavailability of iron". The problems of digestion and absorption clearly constitute one factor. However, between the time iron is absorbed in the gut and the time it is incorporated into hemoglobin, many other metabolic processes are involved. One could be grossly in error if he attributed all changes in hemoglobin concentrations to differences related solely to iron absorption in the gut. Any bioassay procedure for iron that uses hemoglobin concentration as an end-point is open to this error, and one should not be surprised if anomalous results are occasionally encountered. Since most of the change in hemoglobin shown in Figure 1 was systematically related to liver iron concentration, it might be well to consider including this additional measure in any serious attempt to evaluate or understand factors influencing the bioavailability of iron.

Acknowledgements. The authors wish to thank Marie Dent and Julie Doster for their assistance with the early portions of this work and Dr. Marian Wang for her suggestions and encouragement. The work was supported in part by State and Hatch research funds allocated to the Georgia Agricultural Experiment Station.

Literature Cited

1. Caster, W. O.; Parthemos, M. D. Am. J. Clin. Nutr. 1976, 29, 529.
2. Caster, W. O.; Dent, M. Am. J. Clin. Nutr. 1977, 30, 132.
3. Parthemos, M. D. "Biochemical and Physiological Responses of Male, White Rats Fed Common Breakfast Cereals", M.S. Thesis, University of Georgia; Athens, GA, 1974; pp. 172.
4. Cook, J. D.; Finch, C. A. Am. J. Clin. Nutr. 1979, 32, 2115.

5. Caster, W. O.; Doster, J. M. Int. J. Vit. Nutr. Res. 1979, 49, 215.
6. Resurreccion, A. V.; Doster, J. M.; Wang, M.; Caster, W. O. Ga. Sci. J. 1978, 36(2), 65.
7. Resurreccion, A. V.; Doster, J. M.; Wang, M.; Caster, W. O. Sci. Total Environ. 1981, 20, 49.
8. Caster, W. O.; Bleecker, S. J. Nutr. 1975, 105, 308.
9. Yee, H. Y.; Zin, A. Clin. Chem. 1971, 17, 950.
10. Young, D. S.; Hicks, J. M. J. Clin. Path. 1965, 18, 98.
11. Bieri, J. G.; Stoewsand, G. S.; Briggs, G. M.; Phillips, R.W.; Woodard, J. C. J. Nutr. 1977, 107, 1340.
12. Young, G. A.; Anderson, C. K.; Parsons, F. M. Brit. J. Exp. Path. 1973, 54, 241.
13. Passmore, R.; Nicol, B. M.; Rao, M. N. "Handbook on Human Nutritional Requirements", FAO Nutritional Studies No. 28, Rome, 1972; p. 15.
14. Munro, H. N.; et al. "Recommended Dietary Allowances", National Academy of Sciences, Washington, DC, 1980; p. 39.
15. Warner, R. C.; Bruer, L. H. In "Nutrient Requirements of Domestic Animals. No. 10" National Academy of Sciences, Washington, DC, 1972; p. 64.
16. Klevay, L. M. Am. J. Clin. Nutr. 1973, 26, 1060.
17. Caster, W. O.; Doster, J. M. Nutr. Rep. Int., 1979, 19, 773.

RECEIVED July 30, 1982.

7

Effects of Phosphorus-Containing Compounds on Iron and Zinc Utilization

A Review of the Literature

J. L. GREGER

University of Wisconsin, Department of Nutritional Sciences, Madison, WI 53706

A number of investigators have studied the effects of dietary phosphorus on the bioavailability of zinc and iron to animals and human subjects. The results of these studies have not been consistent. Possible reasons for discrepancies among studies include: differences in the types of phosphorus compounds fed; differences in the levels of iron, zinc, ascorbic acid, protein, and calcium fed; and differences in the methods used to assess zinc and iron bioavailability.

Many investigators during the last 50 years have tried to determine whether phosphorus-containing compounds affect the utilization of zinc and iron by animals. These studies have produced divergent and often seemingly inconsistent data. Thus the objectives of this review are: 1) to summarize the results of studies in which the effect of phosphorus on iron and zinc metabolism were investigated; 2) to examine the differences in experimental design and methodology among these studies; and 3) to suggest to what extent these methodological differences account for the differences in the data produced in these studies.

Bioavailability of Iron From Inorganic Compounds Containing Both Phosphorus and Iron

A number of investigators have studied the relative bioavailability of iron from various compounds that contained both iron and phosphorus. Three such salts that have been studied extensively are ferric phosphate, ferric pyrophosphate, and sodium-iron pyrophosphate. All three have been listed as Generally Recognized as Safe (GRAS) in the Code of Federal Regulations and have been added to foods in the United States as iron supplements (1). However, only small amounts of two of these phosphorus-containing salts, ferric pyrophosphate and sodium iron

0097-6156/82/0203-0107$06.00/0

pyrophosphate, have been used as food additives in the United States since 1975. The reasons for the limited use of these two compounds are their limited bioavailability and their cost (2).

Iron in unprocessed ferric phosphate and sodium iron phosphate has extremely low bioavailability as judged by hemoglobin repletion assays with anemic rats and chicks (3-8) (Table I). The absorption of radio-labeled iron from these compounds by non-anemic rats has also been found to be low (9).

Table I: Bioavailability of iron from phosphate salts

	Relative biological value (%)			Absorption of Fe (%)	
Salts	Rats*	Chicks‡	Humans δ	Rats#	Humans**
ferrous sulfate	100	100	100	15.7	2.7-6.6
ferric orthophosphate	12-33	9-18	7	2.9	0.7-1.1
sodium iron pyrophosphate	11-63	2-13	7	1.0	0.3-1.0

*Based on hemoglobin repletion assays (3-6).
‡Based on hemoglobin repletion assays (3).
δBased on change in plasma iron after dose of 50 mg iron (4).
#Based on total body count for ^{59}Fe 1 week after dose (9).
**Based on amount of ^{59}Fe in blood or RBC two weeks after dose (10, 11).

Similarly the bioavailability of iron to human subjects from ferric orthophosphate and sodium iron pyrophosphate has been found to be much lower than the bioavailability of iron from ferrous sulfate (4, 10, 11). The studies with human subjects differed in the manner in which iron bioavailability was judged. Two groups of investigators administered radiotagged iron salts to subjects and measured the levels of ^{59}Fe and ^{55}Fe in the blood or red blood cells two weeks later (10, 11). Pla & Fritz (4) measured the rise in plasma iron levels two hours after a large dose (100 mg iron) of the salt. Despite the differences in methodology in the human and animal studies, the data are fairly consistent. Iron is not very available to men or animals when it is fed to them as an unprocessed inorganic salt of phosphate.

This does not mean that the bioavailability of iron from all compounds containing both phosphorus and iron is low. Wood, et al. (12) and Theuer and his associates (7, 8) have found that the bioavailability of iron from sodium iron pyrophosphate and ferric pyrophosphate was greatly improved when the foods containing these salts were processed with heat and pressure (Table II). Such processing did not, however, improve the bioavailability of iron from ferric orthophosphate or ferrous sulfate. The reason for this effect is not known but sugars in the foods may have formed chelates with the iron that facilitated absorption.

Table II: Effect of processing with heat and pressure on the bioavailability of iron from phosphate salts to rats*

Iron source	Relative biological value	
	Unprocessed	Processed
	%	
ferrous sulfate	100	106
ferric orthophosphate	-10	11
sodium ferric pyrophosphate	14	66‡
ferric pyrophosphate	7	90$^{\delta}$

‡$p<0.05$ difference between unprocessed and processed.
$^{\delta}p<0.01$ difference between unprocessed and processed.
*Reproduced, with permission, from Ref. 12.

Bioavailability of Iron From Organic Compounds Containing Both Phosphorus and Iron

The bioavailability of iron from several organic phosphorus-containing compounds appears to be good. The iron in ferripoly-phosphate protein powder (13) and ferric glycerol phosphate (7, 8) was found to be 92-100% as bioavailable as ferrous sulfate in heme repletion assays with anemic rats and chicks. Morris and Ellis (14) have reported that the iron in monoferric phytate was utilized by rats as well as the iron in ferrous ammonium sulfate. While Lipschitz, et al. (15) have reported that dogs absorbed radio-labelled iron from a small dose (1.5 mg iron) of monoferric phytate one-half as well as they absorbed iron from ferrous sulfate.

Not all organic compounds that contain both phosphorus and iron are good sources of iron. Numerous investigators have demonstrated that the iron in egg yolk was less bioavailable than the iron in reference salts to both men (16, 17) and animals (18-22). This effect of egg yolk on the utilization of iron by animals is due to phosvitin, a glyco-protein in egg yolk (23, 24). This protein contains about 135 phosphoserine groups per molecule. These phosphoryl groups form stable complexes with ferric but less stable complexes with ferrous iron (25).

Effect of Phosphorus on the Bioavailability of Iron and Zinc in the Total Diet

It is important for food scientists to know the bioavailability of iron from various compounds when selecting iron containing compounds to use as food supplements. However, a major concern of nutritionists in regard to the effects of phosphorus-containing compounds on iron and zinc utilization is whether these compounds affect the utilization of the total quantity of iron and zinc in the diet. There are more than 30 different reports in the literature on the effects of dietary phosphorus on zinc and iron utilization. The reported studies have differed in a number of ways. These differences include: 1) the form of dietary phosphorus fed to animals; 2) the species of test animals; 3) the zinc and iron status of the animals; 4) the levels of other dietary factors; and 5) the methods used to assess iron and zinc bioavailability.

Effect of the Forms of Phosphorus. The first factor to be considered in this review is the effect of different forms of phosphorus on trace element utilization. Inorganic phosphorus may occur as simple orthophosphates or condensed phosphates (Figure 1). The condensed or polymeric phosphates include pyrophosphates and polyphosphates. Unfortunately, the nomenclature used to identify most food grade polyphosphates is confusing. For example, sodium hexametaphosphate, which is also called Graham salts and which is a common food additive, generally has a chain length of 10 to 15 phosphorus atoms, not 6 phosphorus atoms as the name implies (26).

Only a few investigators have compared the effects of various forms of phosphorus on zinc and iron utilization by animals. Their results have not been consistent. Mahoney & Hendricks (27) studied the effects of the addition of disodium orthophosphate, sodium pyrophosphate, sodium tripolyphosphate, and sodium metaphosphate to the diets fed to weanling rats. The rats fed orthophosphate, tripolyphosphate, and especially pyrophosphate, absorbed less iron than rats fed the basal diet. Püschner & Bergner (28) also noted that pyrophosphates depressed iron absorption by rats. Hemoglobin levels were depressed in growing rats fed the pyrophosphate and tripolyphosphate in the study by Mahoney & Hendricks. However, neither they nor Dymsza, et al., (29) observed an effect on hemoglobin levels in mature rats. Moreover, neither Mahoney & Hendricks nor Chapman & Campbell (30) noted the inclusion of different forms of phosphorus in the diet affected the level of iron stored in the liver by mature rats. In contrast, Hegsted, et al. (31) noted that an orthophosphate, such as dipotassium orthophosphate, affected iron levels in the livers of rats more than sodium pyrophosphate. However, Hegsted and his associates fed rats a basal diet in which calcium and phosphorus were deleted from the mineral mixture added to the diet while the other investigators fed basal diets with "adequate" levels of phosphorus.

The effect of different forms of phosphorus on zinc utilization appears to be less controversial, perhaps because less has been published on the topic. However, the results of a study by Vohra & Kratzer (32) suggest a possible explanation for the divergent results in the previous studies (Table III). Vohra &

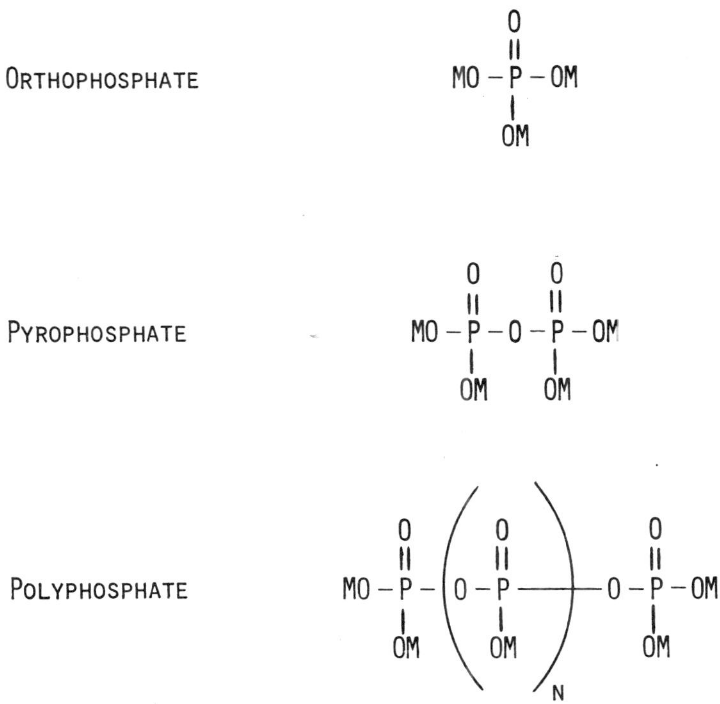

Figure 1. Forms of phosphorus. In these structures, M *represents either hydrogen or a metal ion.*

Kratzer studied the effect of different phosphorus salts on zinc utilization in turkey poults. They fed diets which contained marginal (15 μg/g) levels of zinc. Hence they assumed any factor that inhibited zinc absorption would create a zinc deficient state in the animals and growth would be depressed. They observed if they mixed the zinc and phosphorus salts prior to their addition to the dry diet, most phosphorus salts, especially tripolyphosphate, would depress growth in the turkey poults. However, if they did not mix the zinc and phosphorus salts prior to their addition to the dry diet, the phosphorus salts did not significantly affect growth of the animals.

Table III. Effect of various phosphorus salts on zinc utilization as indicated by weight gain of turkey poults

	Zn & P salts mixed		Zn & P salts not mixed	
Treatment	Trial A‡	Trial B‡	Trial C	Trial D‡
	(g weight gain)			
basal	332^{b}	323^{b}	223	237^{a}
sodium hexametaphosphate	310^{ab}	254^{a}	-	285^{b}
sodium tripolyphosphate	259^{a}	217^{a}	220	252^{ab}
sodium phytate	277^{ab}	241^{a}	203	245^{ab}
sodium acid pyrophosphate	-	-	237	269^{ab}

*Based on tables by Vohra & Kratzer (32).
‡Means in column without the same superscript are significantly ($p<0.01$) different.

The effect of various forms of phosphorus salts on zinc and iron utilization in men have not been assessed. Differences in the cecal flora growth of rats and men could result in differences between the two species in their ability to hydrolyze polyphosphates (33, 34). Thus, at this time it is difficult to speculate whether equal quantities of orthophosphates and polyphosphates in the diet would have different effects on zinc and iron utilization by human subjects.

Effect of Phosphorus on Human Metabolism of Iron and Zinc. Several groups of investigators have examined the effect of orthophosphate salts on iron and zinc utilization by human subjects. Peters, et al. (35) found that the oral administration of sodium orthophosphate salts or dicalcium phosphate with a solution of radiotagged iron chloride and ascorbic acid reduced the retention of ^{59}Fe by human subjects (Table IV). However, Monsen & Cook (36)

Table IV: Effect of phosphorus on the uptake of an oral dose of $^{59}Fe\ Cl_3$ into blood of human subjects*

Additive	Without ascorbic acid	With 50 mg ascorbic acid
	(%)	
None	1.3#	33.2
NaH_2PO_4 and Na_2HPO_4 $^{\delta}$	1.7	1.7
$CaHPO_4$ $^{\delta}$	0.8	1.8

*Based on tables by Peters, et al. (35).
#Mean.
$^{\delta}$1.5 g phosphorus salts.

found that the oral administration of dipotassium phosphate to a meal, rather than just a solution that contained radiotagged iron, did not affect iron absorption of subjects.

The oral administration of inorganic orthophosphate to human subjects may also affect zinc utilization. Pecoud, et al. (37) observed the response of subjects to an oral zinc load test. When fasted subjects were given a large dose (50 mg) of zinc, serum zinc levels rose to 336 μg zinc/100 ml. When subjects were given the same dose of zinc with a meal that contained 468 mg phosphorus or with 480 mg of phosphorus as disodium phosphate, the peak levels of zinc in serum were 98 and 167 μg zinc/100 ml, respectively.

Three other groups of investigators have studied the effects of phosphorus-containing organic compounds on zinc and iron metabolism by human subjects. Snedeker, et al. (38) found that nine subjects absorbed iron and zinc equally well when fed 843 and 2443 mg phosphorus as glycerol phosphate daily. Similarly Spencer et al. (39) noted that the zinc absorption of one subject was constant when he was fed either 800 mg or 1500 mg phosphorus, as glycerol phosphate, daily. Pietreck & Kokot (40) observed no significant changes in serum zinc or iron levels of thirteen subjects fed 15 g of sodium cellulose phosphate daily for nine months.

Effect of Phosphorus on the Metabolism of Iron and Zinc by Animals. These differences in the effects of phosphorus on zinc and iron metabolism are not peculiar to human studies. The differences can certainly be observed in studies with animals. Hegsted, et al. (31) and Buttner & Muhler (41) found that the addition of sodium and potassium orthophosphate salts to diets depressed the utilization of iron by rats, but several groups of investigators have observed that these salts had no effect on iron metabolism by rats (29, 42, 43, 44). Other investigators have observed that the addition of sodium and potassium orthophosphate salts to the diets of steers (45) and chicks (46) depressed iron utilization; still other investigators found these salts had no effect on the iron metabolism of pigs (47), horses (48) or turkeys (49).

Fewer studies have been published on the effects of sodium and potassium orthophosphate salts on zinc metabolism. Four groups of investigators have found these phosphate salts depressed the utilization of zinc by rats (44, 50, 51) and steers (45); three groups have found these phosphate salts had no effect on zinc utilization by pigs (47) and chicks (52, 53).

In general, it does not appear that the different responses of animals to phosphorus in these studies can be attributed to species differences. However, there were many differences in the composition of diets used in these studies. Some of these differences appear to be important.

One way in which the diets varied was in regard to the levels of iron and zinc in the diets. Buttner & Muhler (41) demonstrated that dietary phosphorus levels could only affect iron absorption and hence the amount of iron stored in the liver, if animals were fed diets that contained more than minimal amounts of iron. Similarly Magee & Fu (44) demonstrated with rats that dietary phosphorus levels only affected storage of zinc in the liver if the diets fed the rats contained zinc. Vohra & Kratzer (32) observed a similar phenomenon in turkeys.

Other factors in the diet have also been found to modify the effect of phosphorus on iron and zinc metabolism. One such factor is ascorbic acid. Peters, et al. (35) observed that when human subjects were fed a solution of iron chloride, they absorbed very little iron if ascorbic acid was not present in the solution (Table IV). In fact, if ascorbic acid was not present, absorption of iron was so low it was difficult to tell whether dietary factors, such as phosphorus, affected the absorption of iron. However, ascorbic acid may also counteract the effect of dietary phosphorus on the absorption of nonheme iron. Investigators have demonstrated that the addition of ascorbic acid to a diet counteracted the effect of the phosphoprotein in egg yolk on iron absorption (17, 18).

Dietary protein may also be able to moderate the effect of dietary phosphorus on zinc utilization. Greger & Snedeker (54) observed that human subjects absorbed more zinc when fed a high protein diet with a moderate level of phosphorus than when fed a high protein diet with a high level of phosphorus. This effect of phosphorus was not seen when low levels of protein were fed.

Effect of Phosphorus and Calcium Together on the Bioavailability of Iron and Zinc in the Total Diet

One dietary factor that has been found to exacerbate the effect of phosphorus on zinc and iron utilization is calcium. Several groups of investigators have examined the effect of phosphorus and calcium on iron and zinc metabolism in human subjects. Monsen & Cook (36) fed subjects breakfasts that contained radiotagged iron. The addition of either calcium ($CaCl_2$) or phosphorus (K_2HPO_4) alone to the meal decreased iron absorption, but not significantly (Table V). However, the addition of both calcium ($CaCl_2$) and phosphorus (K_2HPO_4) to the meal significantly depressed iron absorption.

Table V: Influence of the addition of inorganic calcium and inorganic phosphorus to a meal on the absorption of iron by human subjects*

Mineral content of meal		^{59}Fe absorption‡
Ca	P	(%)
(mg)		
24	40	2.2^a
24	414	1.5^a
202	40	1.5^a
202	414	0.6^b

*Based on tables by Monsen & Cook (36).
‡Means with different superscripts are significantly different at the $p<0.005$ level.

Snedeker et al. (38) conducted a metabolic balance study in which each of nine subjects were fed in random order three diets: one diet contained 780 mg calcium and 843 mg phosphorus daily; the second diet contained 780 mg calcium and 2442 mg phosphorus daily; the third diet contained 2382 mg calcium and 2443 mg phosphorus daily (Table VI). The source of the additional calcium was calcium gluconate; the source of the additional phosphorus was glycerol phosphate. The diets were exactly the same in all other respects. Each diet was fed for 12 days. Fecal excretion of iron and zinc was not affected by the addition of just phosphorus to the diet. Fecal excretion of zinc was not affected by the addition of both phosphorus and calcium to the diets. However, fecal iron losses were greater and overall retention of iron was poorer when high levels of both phosphorus and calcium were fed. These differences were not statistically significant. The difference in the data from the study by Monsen & Cook and the data from the study by Snedeker, et al. may reflect the differences in the forms of calcium and phosphorus (inorganic versus organic) fed, the methodology used to measure iron utilization (isotope retention versus metabolic balance), the forms of iron in the diets (all nonheme iron versus a combination of heme and nonheme iron), and the level of ascorbic acid in the diet (undefined or 45 mg per meal).

Table VI: Influence of the addition of calcium gluconate and glycerol phosphorus to diets on the utilization of iron and zinc by human subjects*

diets		iron			zinc		
Ca (mg/day)	P	fecal losses	urinary losses[δ] (mg/day)	balance	fecal losses	urinary losses (mg/day)	balance
780	843	16.7‡	0.1[a]	0.6	10.9	0.8	-1.3
780	2442	16.5	0.1[a]	0.8	11.0	0.8	-1.3
2382	2443	17.9	0.2[b]	-0.4	11.0	0.7	-1.3

*Based on tables by Snedeker, et al. (38).

‡Means (n=9).

δMeans in columns with different superscripts are significantly different at $p<0.05$ level.

Many investigators have studied the combined effect of calcium and phosphorus on iron metabolism on animals. No studies in which phytate was used as the phosphorus source were included in this review (55). In some of the studies included in this review bone meal or a calcium phosphate salt was added to the basal diet. In some, calcium and phosphorus salts were added to the diet separately. All used inorganic sources of calcium and phosphate. In most studies, when both calcium and phosphorus were added to the diet, some parameter of iron status was depressed in rats (44, 56 57,58), in pigs (47,59) in chicks (46,60) and in man (61). Three groups of investigators observed no change in the iron metabolism of horses (48) and cows (62,63) when both inorganic calcium and phosphorus salts were added to diets. One group noted that the addition of bone meal to the diet did not affect hemoglobin levels in normal or anemic rats (64).

Fewer investigators have studied the effect of calcium and phosphorus salts on zinc metabolism in animals than have studied the effect on iron metabolism. The addition of both inorganic calcium and phosphorus to the diet of rats (44,50,51,65) and trout (66) has been found to depress zinc utilization by these animals. However, no changes in zinc metabolism were noted in pigs (47,59) and horses (48) fed high levels of calcium and phosphorus.

Some of the divergence in data from these studies may reflect differences in the methods used to assess iron and zinc status. In several studies hematocrit, hemoglobin and serum iron levels were not affected by dietary calcium and phosphorus levels, but other parameters such as liver or bone iron levels were affected (44,45,47,59). This is not surprising as it is generally recognized that iron stores must be depleted before heme synthesis is impaired (67). Similarly the methods used to assess zinc status in the various studies differed in sensitivity. Less is known about optimal ways to assess zinc status, but generally bone zinc levels are considered to be a more sensitive indicator than serum or liver zinc levels of nutritional status of animals in regard to zinc (68).

In summary, several conclusions can be made on the basis of the studies cited in this review.

1. The bioavailability of iron from unprocessed inorganic phosphate salts is generally low.

2. The relative effects of various forms of dietary phosphorus (i.e. orthophosphates versus polyphosphates) on iron and zinc utilization is not clear and deserves further study.

3. The levels of many other compounds (i.e. ascorbic acid, protein and calcium) in the diet can moderate the effects of phosphorus on zinc and iron utilization. Probably the most important of these factors is calcium. If both inorganic calcium and phosphorus salts are added to a diet, the bioavailability of iron and probably zinc from that diet will be depressed probably.

Acknowledgments

This research was supported by the College of Agricultural and Life Sciences, University of Wisconsin Projects 2398 and 2623 and the Food Research Institute.

Literature Cited

1. Life Science Research Office. "Evaluation of the Health Aspects of Iron and Iron Salts as Food Ingredients." Federation of American Societies for Experimental Biology. Prepared under contract No. FDA 223-75-2004, 1980; 41-43.
2. Lee, K.; Clydesdale, F.M. CRC Critical Rev. in Fd. Sci. & Nutr., 1979, 11, 117-153.
3. Fritz, J.C.; Pla, G.W.; Roberts, T.; Boehne, J.W.; Hove, E.L. J. Agr. Food Chem. 1970, 18, 647-651.
4. Pla, G.W.; Fritz, J.C. Assoc. Off. Anal. Chem. 1971, 54, 13-17.
5. Anderson, T.A.; Kim, I.; Fomon, S.J. Nutr. Metabol. 1972, 14: 355-361.
6. Shah, B.G.; Giroux, A.; Belonje, B. J. Agr. Food Chem. 1979, 27, 845-847.
7. Theuer, R.C.; Kemmerer, K.S.; Martin, W.H.; Zoumas, B.L.; Sarett, H.P., J. Agr. Food Chem. 1971, 19, 555-558.
8. Theuer, R.C.; Martin, W.H.; Wallander, J.F.; Sarett, H.P. J. Agr. Food Chem. 1973, 21, 482-485.
9. Rees, J.M.; Monsen, E.R. J. Agr. Food Chem. 1973, 21, 913-915.
10. Cook, J.D.; Minnick, V.; Moore, C.V.; Rasmussen, A.; Bradley, W.B.; Finch, C.A. Am. J. Clin. Nutr. 1973, 26, 861-872.
11. Rios, E.; Hunter, R.E.; Cook, J.D.; Smith, N.J.; Finch, C.A. Pediatrics 1975, 55, 686-692.
12. Wood, R.J.; Stake, P.E.; Eiseman, J.H.; Shippee, R.L.; Wolski, K.E.; Koehn, V. J. Nutr. 1978, 108, 1477-1484.
13. Jones, S.B.; Kalan, E.B.; Jones, T.C.; Hazel, J.F.; Edmondson, L.F.; Booth, A.N.; Fritz, J.C. J. Agr. Food Chem. 1975, 23, 981-984.
14. Moris, E.R.; Ellis, R. J. Nutr. 1976, 106, 753-760.
15. Lipschitz, D.A.; Simpson, K.M.; Cook, J.D.; Morris, E.R. J. Nutr. 1979, 109, 1154-1160.
16. Chodos, R.B.; Ross, J.F.; Apt, L; Pollycove, M.; Halkett, J.A.E. J. Clin. Invest. 1957, 36, 314-326.
17. Callender, S.T.; Marney, S.R. Jr.; Warner, G.T. Br. J. Haematol. 1970, 19, 657-665.
18. Morris, E.R.; Greene, F.E. J. Nutr. 1972, 102, 901-908.
19. Sherman, W.C.; Elvehjem, C.A.; Hart, E.B. J. Biol. Chem. 1934, 107, 289-295.
20. Narula, K.K.; Wadsworth, G.R. Nutr. Soc. Proc. 1968, 27, 13a.
21. Rose, M.S.; Vahlteich, E.M.; MacLeod, G. J. Biol. Chem. 1934, 104, 217-229.

22. Tompsett, S.L. Biochem. J. 1940, 34, 961-969.
23. Greengard, O.; Sentenac, A.; Mendelsohn, N. Biochem Biophys. Acta 1964, 90, 406-407.
24. Shainkin, R.; Perlmann, G.E. J. Biol. Chem. 1971, 246, 2278-2284.
25. Taborsky, G. J. Biol. Chem. 1980, 255, 2976-2985.
26. Ellinger, R.H. "Phosphates as Food Ingredients", Chemical Rubber Co., Cleveland, Ohio 1972; 3-17.
27. Mahoney, A.W.; Hendricks, D.G. J. Food Sci. 1978, 43, 1473-1476.
28. Püschner, A.; Bergner, H. Arch. Tierernaihr. 1974, 245, 363-374.
29. Dymsza, H.A.; Reussner, G. Jr.; Thiessen, R. Jr. J. Nutr. 1959, 69, 419-428.
30. Chapman, D.G.; Campbell, J.A. Br. J. Nutr. 1957, 11, 127-133.
31. Hegsted, D.M.; Finch, C.A.; Kinney, T.D. J. Exptl. Med. 1949, 90, 147-156.
32. Vohra, P.; Kratzer, F.H. J. Nutr. 1966, 89, 106-112.
33. Zemel, M.B.; Linkswiler, H.M. J. Nutr. 1981, 111, 315-324.
34. Ivey, F.J.; Shaver, K. J. Agr. Food Chem. 1977, 25, 128-130.
35. Peters, T. Jr.; Apt, L.; Ross, J.F. Gastroenterology 1971, 61, 315-322.
36. Monsen, E.R.; Cook, J.D. Am. J. Clin. Nutr. 1976, 29, 1142-1148.
37. Pecoud, A.; Donzel, P.; Schelling, J.L. Clin. Pharmacol. & Therapeut. 1975, 17, 469-474.
38. Snedeker, S.M.; Smith, S.A.; Greger, J.L. J. Nutr. 1982, 112, 136-143.
39. Spencer, H.; Asmussen, C.R.; Holtzman, R.B.; Kramer, L. Am. J. Clin. Nutr. 1979, 32, 1867-1875.
40. Pietrek, J.; Kokot, F. Br. J. Urol. 1973, 45, 136-143.
41. Buttner, W.; Muhler, J.C. Proc. Soc. Exptl. Bio. Med. 1959, 100, 440-442.
42. Fuhr, I.; Steenbock, H. J. Biol. Chem. 1943, 147, 71-75.
43. Grieg, W.A. Br. J. Nutr. 1952, 6, 280-294.
44. Magee, A.C.; Fu, S.C. Nutr. Rep. Intl. 1979, 19, 649-659.
45. Standish, J.F.; Ammerman, C.B.; Palmer, A.Z.; Simpson, C.F. J. Anim. Sci. 1971, 33, 171-178.
46. Sell, J.L. Poultry Sci. 1965, 44, 550-560.
47. Pond, W.G.; Walker, E.F. Jr.; Kirtland, D. J. Anim. Sci. 1978, 46, 686-691.
48. Schryver, H.F.; Hintz, H.F.; Lowe, J.E.; Hintz, R.L.; Harper, R.B.; Reid, J.T. J. Nutr. 1974, 104, 126-132.
49. Sewell, C.E. Jr.; Atkinson, R.L.; Couch, J.R.; Ferguson, T.M. Poultry Sci. 1972, 51, 792-796.
50. Stewart, A.K.; Magee, A.C. J. Nutr. 1964, 82, 287-295.
51. Cabell, C.A.; Earle, I.P. J. Anim. Sci. 1965, 24, 800-804.
52. Pensack, J.M.; Henson, J.N.; Bogdonoff, P.D. Poultry Sci. 1958, 37, 1223-1224.

53. Roberson, R.H.; Schaible, P.J. Poultry Sci. 1960, 39, 837-840.
54. Greger, J.L.; Snedeker, S.M. J. Nutr. 1980, 110, 2243-2253.
55. Cheryan, M. CRC Crit. Rev. Food Sci. & Nutr. 1980, 13, 297-330.
56. Chapman, D.G.; Campbell, J.A. Br. J. Nutr. 1957, 11, 117-126.
57. Day, H.G.; Stein, H.J. J. Nutr. 1938, 16, 525-540.
58. Kletzien, S.W. J. Nutr. 1938, 15 (Suppl), 16.
59. Pond, W.G.; Walker, E.F. Jr.; Kirtland, D. J. An. Sci. 1975, 41, 1053-1056.
60. Waddell, D.G.; Sell, J.L. Poultry Sci. 1964, 43, 1249-1257.
61. Pett, L.B. Fed. Proceed. 1952, 11, 453.
62. Huber, J.T.; Price, N.O. J. Dairy Sci. 1971, 54, 429-432.
63. Steevens, B.J.; Bush, L.J.; Stout, J.D.; Williams, E.I. J. Dairy Sci. 1971, 54, 655-661.
64. Chapman, D.G.; Campbell, J.A. Br. J. Nutr. 1957, 11, 133-137.
65. Heth, D.A.; Becker, W.M.; Hoekstra, W.G. J. Nutr. 1966, 88, 331-337.
66. Ketola, H.G. J. Nutr. 1979, 109, 965-969.
67. Committee on Medical and Biologic Effects of Environmental Pollutants - National Research Council. "Iron" University Park Press, Baltimore, 1979; 79-125.
68. Deeming, S.B.; Weber, C.W. Am. J. Clin. Nutr. 1977, 30, 2047-2052.

RECEIVED June 2, 1982.

Phytate, Wheat Bran, and Bioavailability of Dietary Iron

EUGENE R. MORRIS and REX ELLIS

U.S. Department of Agriculture, Agricultural Research Service, Beltsville Human Nutrition Research Center, Beltsville, MD 20705

Monoferric phytate is the major fraction of iron in wheat bran, and is a highly bioavailable form of dietary iron in contrast to insoluble di- or tetra-ferric phytate. Monoferric phytate equilibrates with the miscible nonheme iron pool of a meal in extrinsic label iron absorption tests. Whole wheat bran depressed absorption by humans of nonheme iron in a meal. Dephytinized wheat bran also inhibited nonheme iron absorption by humans and the inhibition could not be clearly attributed to either the insoluble or soluble fractions of the dephytinized bran. Adult men who consumed 36 g of wheat bran per day had positive iron balances. Iron balance was not increased when dephytinized bran was consumed. The form of ferric phytate must be known to properly explain the effect of phytic acid on iron absorption. The overall meal composition must be considered to evaluate the effect of wheat bran on iron nutrition of humans.

Based on USDA estimates of per capita consumption of wheat flour, one-third of the adult woman's Recommended Dietary Allowance (RDA) for iron could be obtained if we consumed whole wheat products (1). The iron in wheat, however, is thought to be poorly bioavailable to humans, primarily attributable to the effect of phytate. British investigators found that the iron balance of individuals was lower when they ate largely whole meal bread than when they ate bread made with white flour (2). When the test bread made with white flour contained either sodium or ferric phytate, postprandial serum iron rise was depressed (3). They theorized that the phytate present in the brown bread formed an insoluble iron salt and rendered the iron unabsorbable. That theory was supported by the work of Moore et al. (4) at Washington University, who tested the response of anemic individuals administered therapuetic doses of ferric phytate and concluded the iron was poorly absorbed. Hussain et al. (5) found that iron deficiency elicited considerably less enhancement in absorption of wheat iron than of iron from either ferritin or iron salts. They concluded that the mucosal regulation was less effective in this instance because wheat iron was a low bioavailability form of iron.

About a decade ago we began studies to identify the chemical nature of iron in wheat as possibly a first step in devising a means to improve the assimilation of the iron in wheat-based foods. In this communication we will discuss the evidence for our belief that monoferric phytate is the endogenous form of iron in bran, some physical-chemical characteristics of monoferric phytate, and studies in animals and humans of the bioavailability of iron in wheat bran and monoferric phytate.

Monoferric Phytate-Isolation, Identification and Properties

Isolation and identification. The initial isolation of monoferric phytate was from aqueous 1.0-1.2 M ammonium acetate or sodium chloride extracts of wheat bran (6). Approximately 70% of the iron in bran can be extracted in this manner. The extraction of iron is reduced by about 50% if the molarity of the salt solution is reduced to 0.5. Practically no iron can be extracted by water from untreated wheat bran (7). Ammonium sulfate solution, 1M, is also an efficient extraction medium for the iron in wheat bran.

Phytic acid is inositol hexaphosphate. Analysis of the iron containing product isolated from the wheat bran extracts for inositol, phosphorus and iron gave molar ratios of 0.97:6.26:1, respectively, corresponding to a theoretical ratio of 1:6:1 for monoferric phytate. The isolated product exhibited a characteristic absorption spectrum in the 200- to 320-nm range (Figure 1) that corresponded to the spectrum for synthetic monoferric phytate. The Mössbauer spectra (Figure 2) of the iron in wheat bran and of synthetic monoferric phytate also correspond (8).

Solubility characteristics of monoferric phytate. Although a solution of high ionic strength is required to extract monoferric phytate from wheat bran, free monoferric phytate, whether extracted from bran or synthesized, is readily water soluble. We have not tried to determine its maximum solubility in water, but found it insoluble in 50% ethanol:water solution. This later fact enabled its precipitation when prepared from ferric chloride and sodium phytate (6, 9). The product produced by the synthetic method developed by Ellis, described in detail by Lipschitz et al. (9), is a finely divided pale yellow solid.

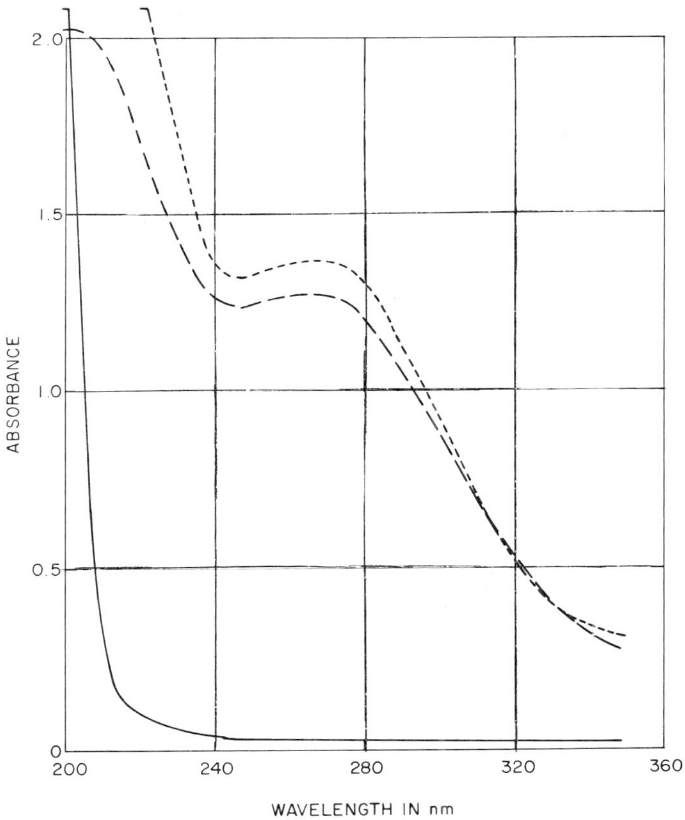

Figure 1. UV absorption spectra of monoferric phytate in 1.2 M ammonium acetate. Solid line, sodium phytate; short dashed lines, monoferric phytate purified from bran; longer dashed lines, synthetic monoferric phytate. (Reprinted, with permission, from Ref. 6. Copyright 1976, American Institute of Nutrition.)

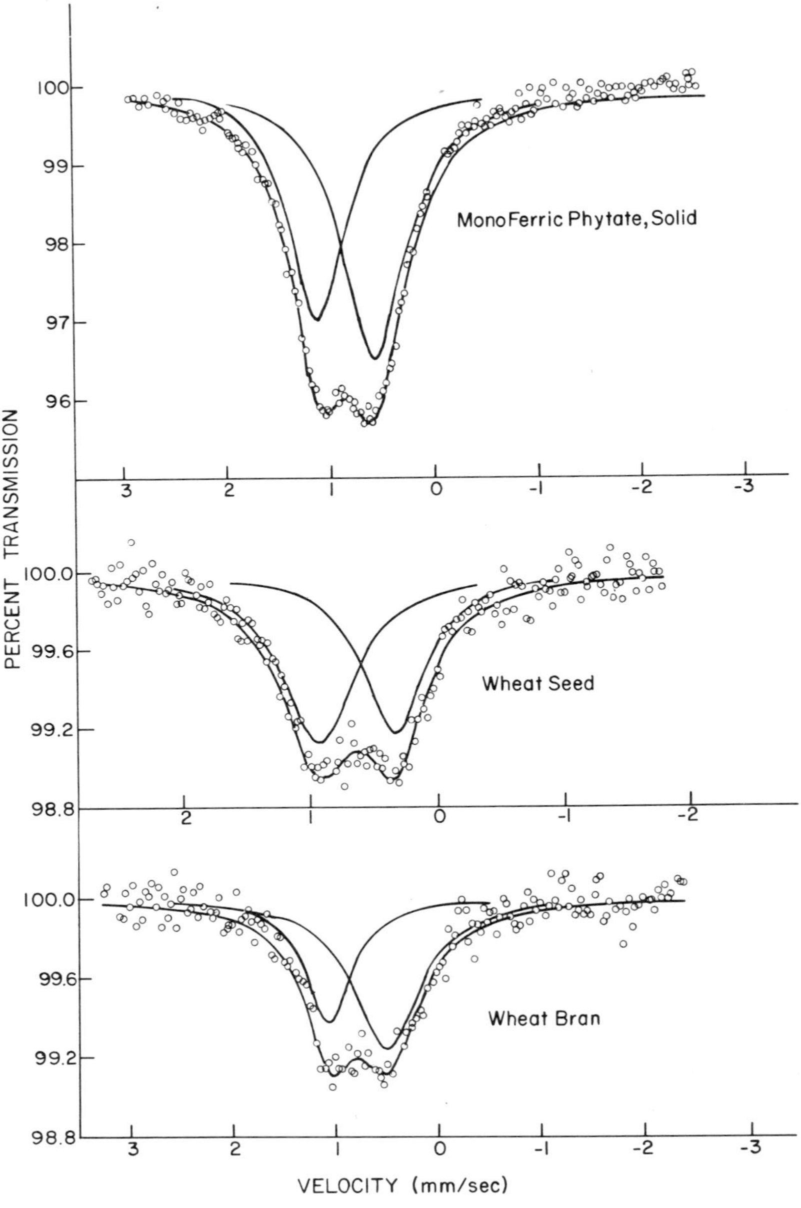

Figure 2. Mössbauer spectra. Top: solid monoferric phytate, 212 mg at 80 K. Center: wheat seeds, 1.54 g at room temperature. Bottom: dissected wheat bran, 9.5 mg at 80 K. All materials enriched in ^{57}Fe. (Reprinted from Ref. 8. Copyright 1980, American Chemical Society.)

Recovery of monoferric phytate subjected to gel-filtration chromatography over a pH range of 1.5 to 10.5 is shown in Figure 3. In 0.05 M buffer recovery was 90% or greater at pH 6.5 to 10.5, but only about 70% at pH 4 to 6, and very low at pH less than 3. Recovery was reduced by at least 50% when 0.5 M sodium chloride was included in the buffer. Further experiments showed that monoferric phytate undergoes a transformation and forms an insoluble product in either 0.1 M HCl or high chloride concentration. In the transformation iron precipitates as insoluble diferric phytate (10). However, 1.3 moles excess of phytate anion prevents this transformation, and the monoferric phytate remains soluble. The presence of excess phytate in the extract made possible the initial extraction in 1 M sodium chloride of monoferric phytate from wheat bran. The transformation does not occur in acetic acid or ammonium acetate solution.

Endogenous form of iron in wheat bran. Because monoferric phytate formed readily in mixtures of sodium phytate and ferric ion, we wondered whether the monoferric phytate in extracts of bran represented an artifact of the extraction procedure rather than represented the chemical form of iron that is endogenous in wheat bran. Two lines of information support our belief that iron exists as monoferric phytate in wheat bran.

First, when Mössbauer spectra were compared between seeds and bran of wheat grown on hydroponic media enriched in ^{57}Fe and synthetic iron phytates (8), the spectra of the seeds and dissected bran (Figure 2) are very similar to the spectrum of solid monoferric phytate. The spectral parameters, quadrupole splitting and isomer shift (Table I), of wheat seeds and bran are identical with those of solid monoferric phytate; all are within the range of those found with high-spin ferric compounds.

Table I. Mössbauer Spectral Parameters of Wheat Seed, Wheat Bran, and Monoferric Phytate[a] (8)

Sample	Quadrupole splitting	Isomer shift
Wheat seeds	0.55	0.76
Wheat bran	0.56	0.77
Monoferric phytate	0.55	0.77

[a]Values are in millimeters per second relative to sodium nitroprusside and were measured at 80 K.

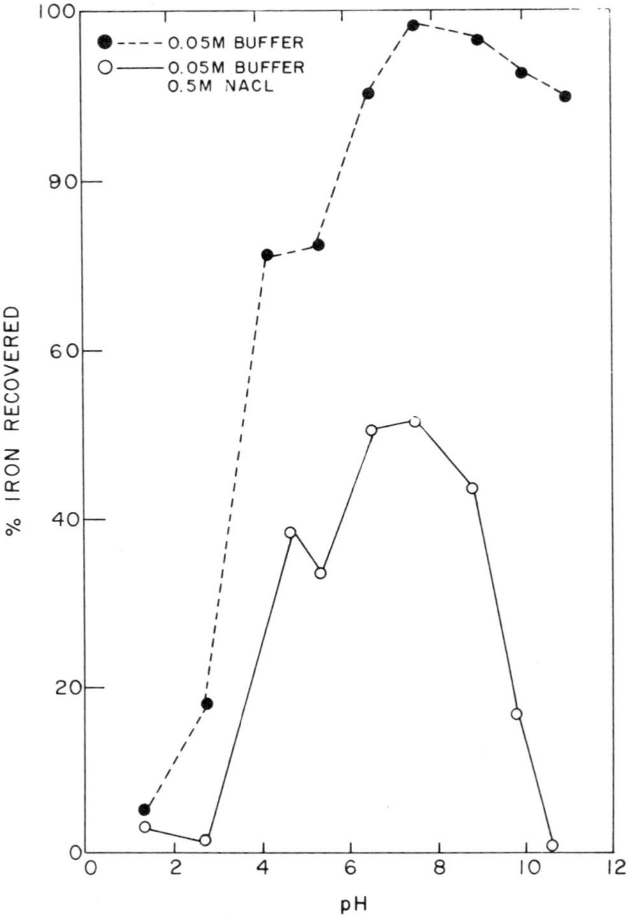

Figure 3. Effect of pH on recovery of monoferric phytate subjected to gel-filtration chromatography. Monoferric phytate samples (40 mg) were chromatographed on a 2 × 50 cm Biogel P-4 column equilibrated with respective buffer.

The parameters indicate that the same iron configuration exists in the wheat seeds and bran and in the monoferric solid. The Mössbauer measurements revealed differences between diferric and monoferric phytate (8).

The second independent line of evidence was derived in the preparation of the low-phytate wheat bran used for zinc bioavailability studies (11). The endogenous phytase of bran was inactivated by autoclaving the dry bran. The autoclaved bran was then extracted with 0.1 M acetate buffer, pH 4.5, at 37°. About 90% of the phytate was extracted by this procedure; phytic acid concentrations in the whole bran and the low-phytate bran were 3.42 and 0.36%, respectively. Only a small amount of iron was present in the 0.1 M acetate extract. The iron in the low phytate product, however, could be extracted as from whole bran by 1.2M ammonium acetate. Gel filtration chromatography of the 1.2 M ammonium acetate extracts of whole and low-phytate bran showed almost equal amounts of monoferric phytate, although total phytate was much less in the extract of the low phytate bran. Thus, even though the bulk of the phytate was extracted by the 0.1 M acetate solution, the iron was not extracted and remained bound in the low-phytate residue. The higher ionic strength solution was required to extract the iron and monoferric phytate was identified as the iron species in the extract. There was a small excess of phytate in the 1.2 M acetate extract of the low phytate residue, but because of the differential extractability, we view the evidence to indicate that monoferric phytate represents the major endogenous fraction of iron in wheat bran.

Bioavailability of Ferric Phytates

Animal studies. In the initial studies (6), a partially purified monoferric phytate prepared from extracts of wheat bran and two synthetic preparations were bioassayed using rats. The hemoglobin depletion-repletion method was used and the relative biological value (RBV) was computed by slope ratio. Compared to the response to ferrous ammonium sulfate as 100, the RBV for the monoferric phytate prepared from wheat bran was 99, and for the two synthetic preparations 101 and 97. The 95% confidence interval for the preparation from wheat bran was 87-111. The iron of monoferric phytate is highly bioavailable to rats.

Ellis and Morris (10) tested di- and tetraferric phytates as dietary iron sources for rats. We harvested diferric phytate from the precipitate that formed when monoferric phytate was suspended in dilute hydrochloric acid and we made tetraferric phytate by adding excess ferric ion to a dilute acid solution of sodium phytate and harvesting the resultant precipitate. After a 3-week feeding period, the hemoglobin responses to monoferric phytate and ferrous ammonium sulfate were about equal (Table II).

Table II. Comparison of Ferric Phytates as Dietary Iron Source for Rats

Iron Source[1]	Hemoglobin[2]
	g/dl
Basal	4.0 ± 0.5^a
$Fe(NH_4)_2(SO_4)_2 \cdot 6H_2O$	10.3 ± 1.2^b
FePhytate	10.6 ± 1.1^b
Fe_2Phytate	5.4 ± 1.1^c
Fe_4Phytate	7.4 ± 0.5^d

[1]Added iron for all diets except basal was 18 µg/g. Diets were fed for 3 weeks. Basal diet contained 6 µg/g of iron.

[2]Mean ± S.E.M. Values with different superscripts are significantly different ($P<0.01$).

However, the hemoglobin response of rats fed a diet that contained diferric phytate was only slightly better than that supported by the low iron basal diet. The response to the tetraferric phytate was intermediate between responses to the di- and monoferric phytate. The bioavailabilities of the iron of the three ferric phytates are markedly different. In another experiment (10), a 60-fold excess of phytic acid as sodium phytate did not depress the ability of monoferric phytate to support hemoglobin formation in growing rats.

Bread is a major wheat-derived food product consumed in the United States. We tested the bioavailability to rats of monoferric phytate either with bread or baked in bread. Either the monoferric phytate or reference iron compound, ferrous ammonium sulfate, was baked in bread at three concentrations of iron. Test diets were formulated by substituting bread for a portion of the glucose monohydrate in the basal iron bioassay diet (see ref. 10 or 11 for details of semipurified diet). Comparable dietary iron concentrations were attained with the same amount of bread in each diet. In addition to diets that contained bread with the iron compound baked in, each compound was added to diets that contained equal amounts of unenriched bread. The bioassay results are shown in Figure 4. The comparison diet (RBV = 100) contained ferrous ammonium sulfate with unenriched bread. There were no differences in the RBV's (calculated by slope ratio) of

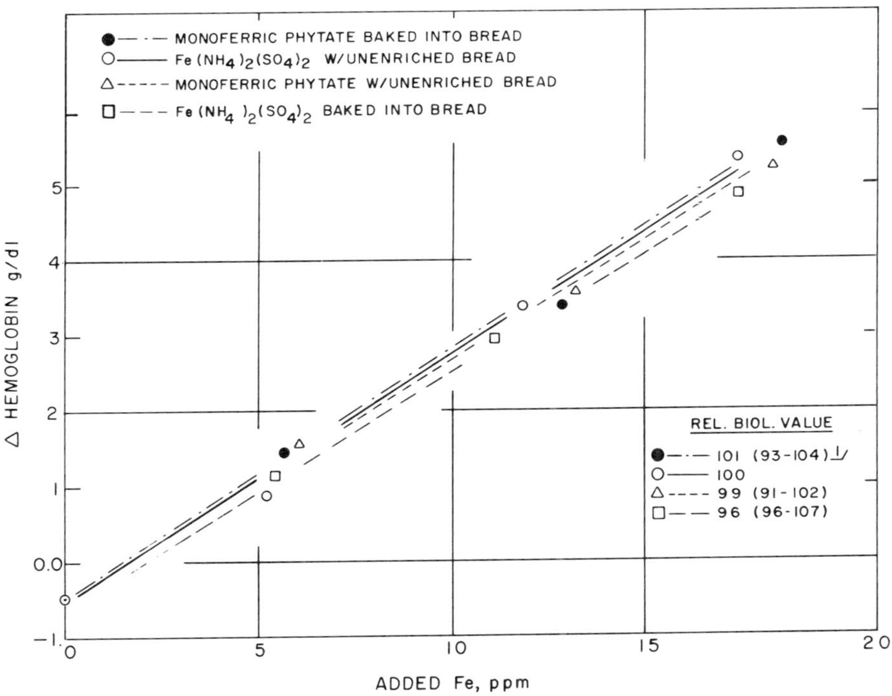

Figure 4. Bioavailability of monoferric phytate baked into bread. Rats were the test species and change in hemoglobin concentration during a 2-week repletion period was bioassay criterion.

the control diet, the reference salt baked into bread or of monoferric phytate, either baked in bread or with unenriched bread. Of the iron in the monoferric phytate-enriched bread, 70% was extracted into 1.2 M ammonium acetate, and the iron chromatographed as monoferric phytate on gel filtration medium.

Ellis and Morris (12) tested the ability of an insoluble calcium-iron-phytate product to support hemoglobin formation in growing rats. The product had an approximate molar composition of Ca_3Fe phytate. After a 3-week feeding period the hemoglobin concentration of rats fed monoferric phytate was 2.7 g/dl greater than for rats fed the insoluble calcium-ferric-phytate product; the difference was significant at $P<0.05$.

Lipschitz et al. (9) tested in dogs the exchangeability of the iron of monoferric phytate and the nonheme iron of a meal. The test meal consisted of the same items, but smaller quantities, as the standard (STD) meal used in human studies of iron absorption (13). The meal was labeled with 0.1 mg iron as $^{59}FeCl_3$ and homogenized; then 0.1 mg iron as ^{55}Fe monoferric phytate was added and the meal was rehemogenized and fed to fasting dogs. Absorption of the isotopes is shown in Figure 5. The mean absorption ratio of the two isotopes was 0.99, indicating that isotopic exchange was complete between the two extrinsic tags. Additional experiments with meals of either high or low bioavailability showed that the iron of monoferric phytate was absorbed to the same extent as the dietary nonheme iron. When either monoferric phytate or ferrous sulfate was administered in solution with no food, the iron of monoferric phytate was absorbed less than half as well as from ferrous sulfate. That result might be explained by the transformation in the absence of food to insoluble diferric phytate in the dogs stomach.

Human studies. Simpson et al. (14) measured absorption by humans of free monoferric phytate from meals of both high and low bioavailability. Absorption was measured by the extrinsic tag method (15). Iron (2 mg) was added to the meals in each pair of absorption tests as either monoferric phytate or $FeCl_3$, each compound was labeled with either ^{55}Fe or ^{59}Fe. The absorption ratio of monoferric phytate to $FeCl_3$ was not significantly different from unity (Table III). The free biological form of iron in wheat bran, monoferric phytate, was no less well absorbed than the dietary nonheme iron in the meals. Absorption of both compounds was several fold greater from the standard (STD) than from the semisynthetic (SS) meal reflecting the relative bioavailability of nonheme iron from the two types of meals.

Table III. Absorption of Extrinsic Labels of Ferric Chloride and Monoferric Phytate by Humans

Semisynthetic Meal		Standard Meal	
$FeCl_3$	FePhy	$FeCl_3$	FePhy
	% of dose[1]		
0.59	0.73	4.73	3.66

$FePhy/FeCl_3$ Absorption Ratio	
SS 1.24(0.96-1.53)[2]	P = 0.24
STD 0.77(0.64-0.94)	P = 0.11

[1]Geometric mean, 9 subjects.
[2]Mean ratio (± SE).

Bioavailability of Iron in Wheat, Wheat Fractions and Wheat Foods

Animal studies. A series of bioassays in our laboratory showed that in its bioavailability to rats the iron in wheat and its major milling fraction is equivalent to the iron of ferrous ammonium sulfate. Both prophylatic and therapeutic hemoglobin responses were tested and the 95% confidence interval showed no significant difference from ferrous ammonium sulfate (16). However, the RBV of iron in some wheat-based food products has significantly lower bioavailability. In three of four different bioassays of whole wheat bread, the RBV differed significantly from ferrous ammonium sulfate (16).

Table IV presents the RBV for the iron of three breakfast cereals not fortified with iron. The two ready-to-eat cereals were sources of highly bioavailable iron, but the instant cereal was significantly lower in bioavailability than the reference salt. We have not studied the chemical nature of iron in commercially available wheat based foods. The iron that remains in the residue of 1.2 M ammonium acetate extracted wheat bran was only 71% as bioavailable as the extracted monoferric phytate (6), but the iron of enzymatically dephytinized wheat bran, which may be complexed with amino acids, is highly bioavailable (11).

Table IV. Relative Biological Value to Rats of Iron in Wheat Breakfast Cereals

Cereal Type[1]	RBV[2]	95% Confidence Limits
Ready to eat, whole wheat	100	81-121
Ready to eat, bran	89	74-107
Instant whole wheat, to be served hot	72	55-90

[1]Not fortified with iron.

[2]Relative biological value, percentage based on response to $Fe(NH_4)_2(SO_4)_2 \cdot 6H_2O$ = 100.

Human studies. A set of experiments, conducted in cooperation with the Division of Hematology, University of Kansas Medical Center, attempted to delineate the role of phytate on absorption of iron from wheat bran by humans (14). Absorption of nonheme iron was measured by the extrinsic tag method. The first pair of absorption tests demonstrated that, when muffins contained 6 g of wheat bran, the absorption of nonheme iron from a meal of 2 muffins, a milkshake and beef patty was markedly reduced. In a second pair of tests with the same subjects the same level of inhibition by bran was observed from a meal of 2 muffins and milkshake with 100 mg of ascorbic acid, even though the level of absorption was more than doubled. In each pair of tests, the ratio of absorption with/without bran in the muffins was 0.49 which differed significantly from unity ($P<0.001$). The second experiment compared plain muffins to muffins that contained either dephytinized bran or bran that had been lyophylized, or untreated bran in a meal with a milkshake plus ascorbic acid. Absorption was significantly greater ($P<0.05$) with dephytinized bran than with untreated bran (Table V) but all three types of bran, compared to no bran, significantly ($P<0.01$) inhibited absorption of dietary nonheme iron. Wetting of the bran and lyophylization without changing the phytate content appeared to decrease the inhibition of iron absorption by the bran (B vs C in Table V). The meal with dephytinized bran contained the same amount of total phosphorus as the meal with the untreated bran, but most was present as phosphate rather than phytate phosphorus. Therefore, in a third experiment we separated dephytinized bran into soluble and insoluble fractions and tested the effect of each on absorption of dietary nonheme iron. The whole dephytinized bran inhibited iron absorption

Table V. Dephytinized Wheat Bran and Absorption of Nonheme Dietary Iron by Humans [1]

No Bran (A)	Untreated Bran (B)	Lyophlized Bran[2] (C)	Dephytinized Bran[3] (D)
	% of dose		
2.43	0.99	1.29	1.37
B/A	0.41 (0.37-0.46)[4]	P< 0.0001	
C/A	0.53 (0.44-0.65)	<0.01	
D/A	0.56 (0.46-0.69)	<0.01	
B/C	0.77 (0.63-0.93)	0.10	
B/D	0.73 (0.63-0.84)	<0.05	

[1]Meal was milkshake w/100 mg ascorbic acid and 2 muffins. Bran muffins contained 6 g of respective bran per muffin. Ten subjects.

[2]Bran was immersed in water, immediately frozen then freeze dried, phytate concentration equaled untreated bran, 139 mg phytic acid per meal.

[3]Dephytinized by endogenous phytase. Phytic acid per meal was reduced to 9 mg.

[4]Mean ratio ($\pm$ 1 SE).

(Table VI), but the degree of inhibition was less than that in the previous set of tests. Compared to absorption from the meal without bran, iron absorption with the insoluble fraction was greater, and that with the soluble fraction less, but neither differed significantly from the no bran meal. Absorption was almost the same with the soluble fraction and the whole dephytinized bran. However, with the insoluble fraction, which was very low in phosphate ion, absorption was significantly greater than with either the soluble fraction or the whole dephytinized bran, both of which contained phosphate ion. The amount of neutral detergent fiber in the insoluble fraction meal was almost the same as in the whole dephytinized bran meal, but the soluble fraction meal was low in neutral detergent fiber

Table VI. Effect of Soluble and Insoluble Fractions of Dephytinized Wheat Bran on Absorption of Dietary Nonheme Iron by Humans [1]

No Bran	Dephytinized Bran[2]		
	Whole	Insoluble	Soluble
(A)	(B)	(C)	(D)
% of Dose			
3.02	2.23	3.22	2.43

B/A	0.74 (0.62-0.88)[3]	P< 0.053
C/A	1.07 (0.91-1.26)	0.35
D/A	0.81 (0.69-0.95)	0.10
C/B	1.45 (1.21-1.72)	<0.05
D/B	1.09 (0.90-1.33)	0.33
D/C	0.76 (0.61-0.85)	<0.05

[1]Meals consisted of milkshake with 100 mg ascorbic acid and 2 muffins, bran muffins contained 12 g dephytinized bran or equivalent per meal. Eighteen subjects.

[2]Dephytinized enzymatically by endogenous phytase.

[3]Mean ratio ($\pm$ 1 SE).

content. The work with the University of Kansas investigators indicates that whole wheat bran inhibits the absorption of dietary nonheme iron, but the inhibiting action apparently does not reside in the monoferric phytate or in the fiber alone. Interaction or synergistic action between fiber and phytate is a possibility.

We conducted a metabolic balance study, in conjunction with the Human Study Facility at Beltsville, to compare mineral balance of humans consuming whole bran or dephytinized bran continuously over several weeks. Results of this study have been published in part (17, 18, 19), and the results for iron will be summarized here. Ten adult men consumed menus that repeated in cycles of 5 days. The food items were usual foods consumed in the United States, no semipurified preparations. Each meal included two bran muffins that contained 6 g each of either whole bran or dephytinized bran (36 g of bran consumed each day). The bran was milled from a single lot of hard red spring wheat and one-half was dephytinized by action of the endogenous phytase. The mean iron intake was 18.2 mg per day, approximately one-third in the muffins. Phytic acid intakes were 2.0 and 0.2 g per day, respectively, when whole bran muffins or dephytinized bran muffins were consumed, but there was no difference in neutral detergent fiber intakes, 17 g per day.

Each type of bran muffin was consumed for 15 days, 3 repeats of the 5-day menu cycle. One-half of the subjects (subjects 1-5) first consumed whole bran muffins then dephytinized bran muffins and one-half (subjects 6-10) consumed them in the reverse sequence. Stools were collected and pooled the first 5 days and stools and urine were collected and pooled for the last 10 days. Apparent absorption (intake minus excretion in feces) was calculated for the 5- and 10-day periods, but balances were calculated only for the 10 day period.

The mean daily iron balance for each subject when consuming each type of bran is shown in Fig. 5. Iron balance for subjects 1-5 was slightly more positive when they consumed the dephytinized bran muffins, but for subjects 6-10, balance was 2 mg/day more positive when they consumed the whole bran muffins. The mean iron balance for all subjects was almost 0.9 mg/day more positive during the consumption of whole bran muffins, but the most positive balances were observed during the second balance period regardless of the sequence in which the bran types were eaten. Apparent iron absorption values (Table VII) were more positive for the last 10 days than for the first 5 days each type of muffin was consumed and tended to be negative the first 5 days whole bran muffins were consumed regardless of the sequence. Subjects 1-5 tended to have more positive values of apparent absorption as the study progressed. However, subjects 6-10, who consumed dephytinized bran muffins followed by whole bran muffins, excreted on the average more iron in the feces than they consumed for the first 5 days they consumed whole bran muffins.

Discussion

We believe the endogenous form of iron in wheat bran is monoferric phytate. The differential extractability from bran of monoferric phytate versus the bulk of the phytate and the comparable Mössbauer parameters of the iron in synthetic mono-

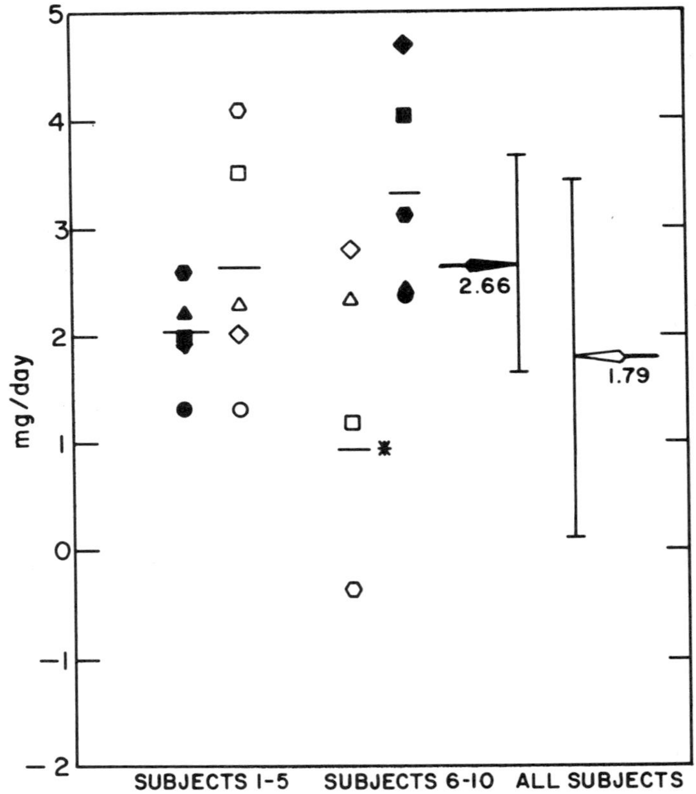

Figure 5. Iron balance of adult men consuming 36 g of whole wheat bran or dephytinized bran per day. The arrows and vertical bars (all subjects) represent mean ± 1 SD. Balances are for the last 10 days of a 15-day period in which each type of bran muffin was consumed. Solid symbols, with phytate; open symbols, without phytate.

Table VII. Effect of Type of Bran Muffin on Apparent Absorption of Iron by Adult Men

Whole Bran Muffin		Dephytinized Bran Muffin	
5 days	10 days	5 days	10 days
	mg/day[1]		
	Subjects 1-5[2]		
-3.0 ± 1.1	2.2 ± 0.4	1.3 ± 2.5	2.8 ± 1.1
	Subjects 6-10[2]		
-0.3 ± 2.5	3.5 ± 0.9	0.0 ± 1.6	1.1 ± 1.8
	All Subjects		
-1.6 ± 1.6	2.9 ± 0.7	0.7 ± 1.6	2.0 ± 1.1

[1]Intake minus fecal excretion, means ± SD, 10 subjects total.

[2]Subjects 1-5 consumed whole bran muffins the first 15 days then consumed dephytinized bran muffins. Subjects 6-10 consumed the muffins in the reverse sequence.

ferric phytate and in seeds or bran support this conclusion. The solubility of monoferric phytate in water likely explains the high bioavailability of the iron from monoferric compared to iron from the relatively insoluble di or tetraferric phytates. Possibly the ferric phytates used by Moore et al. (4) for humans and by Bremner and Dalgarno (20) for calves were mixtures of all possible ferric phytates, but were predominately insoluble forms and the iron was poorly bioavailable. We found the iron of an insoluble calcium ferric phytate product to be of low bioavailability. Sharpe et al. (21) added sodium phytate and ferric chloride labeled with radioiron to milk and found that the radioiron was poorly absorbed by adolescent boys. Possibly insoluble calcium ferric phytate formed in that experiment.

Approximately 70% of the monoferric phytate baked into bread could be recovered in extracts of the bread. We have not tested the bioavailability or the chemical form of iron when an iron salt and sodium phytate are baked into bread as was done by McCance et al. (3). If an insoluble ferric phytate of any ion composition was formed, we would expect the iron to be poorly bioavailable. Hussain and Patwardhan (22) did not specify whether they added sodium phytate to the food during preparation or administered it orally when young men ate the meals in their study using a vegetarian menu. They found decreased iron balance when the percentage of phytate phosphorus to total phosphorus was increased from 8 to 40 by addition of sodium phytate.

Phytase is present in the rat intestine (23, 24) and the potential to hydrolyze dietary phytate has been suggested as the explanation for the rat's ability to utilize iron in wheat. Phytase activity is also found in the mucosa of the chicken, calf and man (26), but the quantitative aspects have not been examined. In rats, the activity is evidently highly dependent upon calcium content of the diet (26) and very probably of other cations such as zinc and magnesium that will complex with phytate. Hunter (27) concluded that high levels of sodium phytate in the diet of rats does not inhibit utilization of dietary iron, and this agrees with our observations. The existence in wheat of monoferric phytate, a highly bioavailable form of iron, seems a more likely explanation of the rats ability to utilize the iron. Also, the stabilizing action of excess phytate on the stability of monoferric phytate may actually aid in the utilization of iron of bran. The form of iron in other cereals and legumes is uncertain. The iron in soybeans was well utilized by rats and may contain a fraction of the iron as monoferric phytate (28). Welch and Van Campen (29) determined that ^{59}Fe from mature soybeans was more bioavailable than that from immature seeds even though the mature seeds contained approximately three times as much phytic acid. Peas and lima beans were better sources of bioavailable iron than were navy beans (30), but the chemical nature of the iron is uncertain and phytate was not determined. Sathe and Krishnamurthy (31) found poor utilization by rats of iron from unpolished as compared to polished rice.

Binding of nutritionally important cations to dietary fiber has recently been introduced as a possible cause for poor utilization by humans of iron from diets high in vegetables and unrefined cereals. Reinhold et al. (32) and Ismail-Beigi et al. (33) have demonstrated that the fiber component of wheat bread and bran binds iron even after the phytate has been extracted by dilute acid. In our study, the water-insoluble fraction (containing most of the neutral detergent fiber of the bran) of enzymatically dephytinized wheat bran did not inhibit, whereas the soluble portion (almost devoid of neutral detergent fiber) did inhibit absorption of nonheme iron. The latter fraction was high in phosphate which has been demonstrated to inhibit iron absorption by humans (34). Also, ferric orthophosphate iron is poorly absorbed by humans (35). There was no difference in neutral detergent fiber analysis of the two types of bran muffins consumed in our metabolic balance study. The high level of phosphate might have influenced iron balance when the dephytinized bran muffins were consumed. Thus, we have not conclusively demonstrated either that phytate-free bran does not depress iron balance or that a phytate-fiber complex binds iron and inhibits iron absorption.

Two factors, high intakes of total iron and of ascorbic acid, may have contributed to the relatively high positive iron balances when the whole bran muffins were consumed. Iron intakes averaged 180% of the recommended dietary allowance for adult men (36) and even without the bran would have averaged 120%. Thus, if high iron intake was a determinant of the magnitude of the balance, the contribution of wheat bran to total iron consumed in American diets is an important consideration in iron nutrition. Apte and Venkatchalain's (37) subjects required more than 16 mg of iron per day to maintain a clearly positive iron balance when they consumed a high phytate (40% of total phosphorus as phytate phosphorus) cereal based diet. Ascorbic acid enhances absorption of dietary nonheme iron (38). The menus consumed in our metabolic balance study included citrus juice once or twice each day and overall were generous in ascorbic acid. The ascorbic acid content coupled with the frequency of beef, poultry or pork in the meals would class most of the meals in the high iron bioavailability category (39). This also may have been an important determinant for the magnitude of the iron balances.

Summary

The major fraction of iron in wheat bran is monoferric phytate, which is soluble and equilibrates with the miscible dietary nonheme iron pool of a meal. The di- and tetra-ferric phytates are much less soluble than monoferric phytate and probably do not equilibrate with the miscible nonheme iron pool of a meal. Bioavailability studies using either ferric phytate or sodium phytate must be evaluated in light of the form of ferric phytate or whether an insoluble ferric phytate may have been produced in the food. Wheat bran depresses absorption of dietary nonheme iron by humans. On the basis of available evidence, that effect of wheat bran cannot be unequivocally attributed to either the phytate or fiber component alone and might be influenced by interactions between the fiber, phytate and iron in the whole bran. Adult men maintained adequate positive iron balance when they consumed 36 g of whole bran each day in meals that generally classify as high in bioavailability for iron. Total iron intake and other meal components must be considered in assessing the impact of wheat bran on iron nutrition.

Literature Cited

1. Morris, E.R. Baker's Dig. 1974, 48, 32.
2. Widdowson, E.M.; McCance, R.A. Lancet 1942, I, 588.
3. McCance, R.A.; Edgecombe, C.N., Widdowson, E.M. Lancet 1943, II, 126.
4. Moore, C.V.; Minnich, V.; Dubach, R. J. Amer. Dietet. Assoc. 1943, 19, 841.
5. Hussain, R.; Walker, R.B.; Layrisse, M.; Clark, P.; Finch, C.A. Amer. J. Clin. Nutr. 1965, 16, 464.
6. Morris, E.R.; Ellis, R. J. Nutr. 1976, 106, 753.
7. Morris, E.R.; Greene, F.E.; Marsh, A.C. In: Hoekstra, W.G.; Suttie, J.W.; Ganther, H.E.; Mertz, W. "Trace Element Metabolism in Animals-2"; University Park Press, Baltimore, 1974; p. 506.
8. May, L.; Morris, E.R.; Ellis, R. J. Agric. Food Chem. 1980, 28, 1004.
9. Lipschitz, D.A.; Simpson, K.M.; Cook, J.D.; Morris, E.R. J. Nutr. 1979, 109, 1154.
10. Ellis, R.; Morris, E.R. Nutr. Rep. Int. 1979, 20, 739.
11. Morris, E.R.; Ellis, R. J. Nutr. 1980, 110, 2000.
12. Ellis, R.; Morris, E.R. Nutr. Res., in press.
13. Cook, J.D.; Monsen, E.R. Amer. J. Clin. Nutr. 1975, 28, 1289.
14. Simpson, K.M.; Morris, E.R.; Cook, J.D. Amer. J. Clin. Nutr. 1981, 34, 1469.
15. Layrisse, M.; Martinez-Torres, C.; Cook, J.D.; Walker, R.; Finch, C.A. Blood 1973, 41, 333.
16. Morris, E.R.; Ellis, R. Baker's Dig. 1976, 50, 28.
17. Morris, E.R.; Ellis, R. Cereal Foods World, 1979, 24, 461 (Abstr.).
18. Morris, E.R.; Ellis, R.; Steele, P.; Moser, P. Fed. Proc. 1980, 39, 787 (Abstr.).
19. Morris, E.R.; Ellis, R.; Steele, P.; Moser, P. In: Hemphill, D.D. ed., "Trace Substances in Environmental Health-XIV", University of Missouri-Columbia 1980, p. 103.
20. Bremner, I.; Dalgarno, A.C. Br. J. Nutr. 1973, 29, 229.
21. Sharpe, L.M.; Peacock, W.C.; Cooke, R.; Harris, R.S. J. Nutr. 1950, 41, 433.
22. Hussain, R.; Patwardhan, V.N. Ind. J. Med. Res. 1959, 47, 676.
23. Patwardhan, V.N. Biochem. J. 1937, 31, 560.
24. Pileggi, V.J. Arch. Biochem. Biophys. 1959, 80, 1.
25. Bitar, K.; Reinhold, J.G. Biochim. Biophys. Acta 1972, 268, 442.

26. Nahapetian, A; Young, V.R. J. Nutr. 1980, 110, 1458.
27. Hunter, J.E. J. Nutr. 1981, 111, 841.
28. Ellis, R.; Morris, E.R. Cereal Chem. 1981, 58, 367.
29. Welch, R.M.; VanCampen, D.R. J. Nutr. 1975, 105, 253.
30. Morris, E.R.; Marsh, A.C. Fed. Proc. 1973, 32, 923 (Abstr.).
31. Sathe, V.; Krishnamurthy, K. Ind. J. Med. Res. 1953, 41, 453.
32. Reinhold, J.G.; Ismail-Beigi, F.; Faradji, B. Nutr. Rep. Int. 1975, 12, 75.
33. Ismail-Beigi, F.; Faraji, B.; Reinhold, J.G. Am. J. Clin. Nutr. 1977, 30, 1721.
34. Peters, T.; Apt, L.; Ross, J.F. Gastroent. 1971, 61, 315.
35. Cook, J.D.; Minnich, V.; Moore, C.V.; Rasmussen, A.; Bradley, W.B.; Finch, C.A. Am. J. Clin. Nutr. 1973, 26, 861.
36. National Research Council, Recommended Dietary Allowances, National Academy of Sciences, Washington, DC, 1980.
37. Apte, S.V.; Venkatachalam, P.S. Ind. J. Med. Res. 1962, 50, 516.
38. Lynch, S.R.; Cook, J.D. in Levander, O.A.; Cheng, L. "Micronutrient Interactions: Vitamins, Minerals and Hazardous Elements", Ann. N.Y. Acad. Sci. 1980, 355, 32.
39. Monsen, E.R.; Hallberg, L.; Lyrisse, M.; Hegsted, D.M.; Cook, J.D.; Mertz, W.; Finch, C.A. Am. J. Clin. Nutr. 1978, 31, 134.

RECEIVED June 2, 1982.

9

Dietary Fiber and the Bioavailability of Iron

JOHN G. REINHOLD

University of Guadalajara, Faculty of Veterinary Medicine and Animal Science, Center for the Study of Nutrition, Apdo. Postal 406-1, Guadalajara, Jalisco, México.

Iron II combines with several components of dietary fiber to form complexes that are stable between pH 6.0 and 7.0. Iron so bound is released as the pH falls below 6.0, release becoming complete near pH 1.0. Binding is inhibited by ascorbate, citrate, cysteine, EDTA and phytate in low concentrations. The various components of dietary fiber differ in affinity for iron. Dietary fiber from different sources, e.g., wheat and maize, have differing capabilities for binding iron. Increased consumption of dietary fiber or fiber-rich foods tends to impair iron absorption. Impairment is best demonstrated if single fiber sources are used, and when the amount in the diet is 10 % or more. Consumption of large amounts of wheaten fiber by human subjects has been associated with increased fecal losses of iron and decreased iron balances. Concentrations of iron in serum tend to decrease. The presence of inhibitors of iron binding in diets may explain, in part, differences in response to fiber. Calculation of the amount of iron sequestered indicates that only when dietary fiber intakes are quite high will iron binding seriously interfere with absorption of iron. However, other actions of fiber contribute to impairment of iron availability.

0097-6156/82/0203-0143$06.00/0

Dietary fiber may interfere with iron absorption by several actions. The increase in weight and bulk of undigested residues in the gut that follows intake of fiber in increased amounts leads to decreased transit times and increased frequency of defecation. Fecal weight increases. The time of contact between villi and iron decreases with lessened opportunity for absorption. Eastwood and Kay (1) have likened the behavior of dietary fiber to that of a sponge with both fibrous and amorphous properties. Iron may enter the pores of the fiber to become compartmented and spatially hindered from making close contact with the mucosa. The increased fecal bulk combined with the abrasiveness of dietary fiber may combine to increase losses of iron by the sloughing of mucosal epithelium, normally a major pathway for excretion of iron. Fiber provides a matrix for the gut flora and so may stimulate its growth. With increased incorporation of iron into bacterial cells, iron so diverted is no longer available for absorption. The major components of dietary fiber, cellulose and the hemicelluloses, form complexes with iron (2,3). Dietary fiber may promote the conversion of iron II to iron III in some circumstances. Such a conversion would tend to decrease iron availability.

Dietary fiber includes cellulose and lignin which together comprise the acid-detergent fiber (ADF)(4) fraction; the hemicelluloses, a complex group with a polymerized xylose framework with arabinose, mannose, galactose, glucose, rhamnose, glucuronic and galacturonic acid substitutions and differing degrees of branching; and pectin, a mixture of methyl-esterified galacturonan, galactan, and araban. Cereal grains contain little pectin. Total dietary fiber is conveniently isolated and measured as neutral detergent fiber (NDF) which includes the foregoing components (5,6). In addition to the dietary fiber occurring naturally in foods, nondigestible polysaccharides from seaweeds and other sources, including gums, are included and become important because of their widespread use as food additives. For detailed information about the composition of dietary fiber see (6,7,8).

Evidence that dietary fiber interfered with absorption of bivalent metals by the intestine was first obtained in connection with studies of human zinc deficiency in Iran. Human subjects who consumed purified phytate exhibited smaller fecal losses of zinc and calcium than they did when they ate equivalent amounts of phytate in the form of unleavened wheaten whole meal flat breads that are the staple food in rural Iran (9). Bread components other than phytate were examined for their ability to bind metals. Fiber, protein and starch of wheat formed stable complexes with zinc and calcium, and later iron was found to share this behavior. The metals combined with protein or wheat starch, however, were released during digestion with peptidases and amylases (2,10). By contrast dietary fiber, being resistant to digestive secretions, retained bound metal intact. Removal of phytate, which had in the past been held to be the main source of metal complexation by bread, did not decrease but tended to enhance the binding of the metal (2). Further doubt about the role of phytate as the metal binding agent of breads was introduced by the absence of a close relationship between the destruction of phytate by action of leaven and the solubility of zinc (11). Subsequently, studies by Ismail-Beigi et al.(3) showed that cellulose from some sources, certain cellulose derivatives, and hemicelluloses prepared from wheat bran shared the ability to bind iron and zinc. Camire and Clydesdale (12) recently described differences in the iron binding capability of several cellulose preparations.

Affinity of Dietary Fiber Preparations for Iron

Uptake of iron II by NDF suspended in solutions of the composition described below and buffered at pH 6.4 is rectilinear up to iron concentrations of about 1.5 ug/ml (13). Above the latter concentration, the iron becomes unstable and the results erratic. The quantity of iron bound by NDF of wheat exceeded that bound by the NDF of maize by about 25 % . Binding by ADF and by cellulose (finely divided filter paper or absorbent cotton) were equal and about half of the amount of iron bound by wheat NDF. For measurement of binding, 20 mg of fiber were suspended in 10 ml of a solution containing 7.5 g of NaCl, 5.0g of D-glucose,

0.3 g of KCl, sodium acetate 1.0 mMol, imidazole 0.5 mMol, HCl, 0.2 mMol, ascorbic acid 0.28 mMol and iron as $FeSO_4$ 0.0129 mMol per liter. pH was adjusted to 6.40 ± 0.05[4]. After equilibration for 30min, the fiber was removed by centrifugation and iron measured in the solution with the aid of sulfonated bathophenanthroline (13).

When iron bound by fiber at several iron concentrations was plotted against the ratio: bound iron/free iron, straight lines resulted. Intercepts with the axis for bound iron yielded coefficients of binding for wheat NDF, 0.39; maize NDF, 0.30; maize or wheat ADF, 0.24; cellulose 0.22 mg iron/g fiber (13).

Monnier et al (14) using conditions quite different from those described above, found no iron to be bound by cellulose, but did find that pectin bound iron strongly. Water-and alkali-soluble hemicelluloses prepared from rice bound iron (Mod et al, 15). Copper and zinc were also bound. The metals were released by hemicellulase and peptidase action. These hemicellulose isolates included considerable amounts of digestible protein and consequently do not conform to the concept of fiber as a non-digestible residue. However, close associations of fiber and protein do occur and their implications for fiber behavior must be recognized Mod et al (15) assign a role to fiber bound protein in binding of metals. Thompson and Weber (16) observed that ion exchange properties of dietary fiber depended upon method of preparation.

Effect of pH upon Binding of Iron by Dietary Fiber

Binding of iron by dietary fiber approaches a maximum as pH approaches 7.0 (13). It is minimal in the neighborhood of pH 1.0 Thompson and Weber (16) and Reilly (17) showed that the effects of pH were reversible over the range 1.0 to 7.0. Camire and Clydesdale (12) found a marked change in binding of iron by cellulose to occur between pH 5.0 and 6.0 after boiling, and by lignin after toasting, but not by toasted or boiled wheat bran. Working with NDF prepared by the method of Robertson and Van Soest (5), Reinhold et al (13) showed that binding of iron traced a sinusoidal path between pH 5.0 and 7.0 with a midpoint at about pH 5.8. NDF from wheat and maize described identical curves which differed in height because of difference in affinity for iron between the two. Wheat and maize brans behaved like their NDFs. The locations and configurations of the curves were not altered by removal of phytate. Binding of iron by cellulose or ADF preparations also decreased markedly between pH 7.0 and 5.0 but to a lesser extent than did the NDFs (13).

Inhibition of Iron Binding

Binding of iron by dietary fiber is strongly inhibited by ascorbic acid, citrate, cysteine, EDTA or phytate in concentrations as low as 100 μMols/Liter (13). The inhibitors have the common property of being able to form soluble complexes with iron. The decarboxylic amino acids and their amides inhibit binding moderately as do lysine and histidine. Other amino acids either do not interfere with binding of iron fiber or do so only weakly. Calcium (as acetate) and phosphate act as moderate inhibitors. The detergents sodium lauryl sulfonate or cetyltrimethylammonium bromide had no effect on iron binding by fiber (13).

Stability of Fiber-Bound Iron in Presence of Intestinal segments

Segments of rat intestine readily absorb iron from an iron-containing saline glucose solution similar to that described above. The up-take of iron by the segments is decreased significantly by NDF or nondigestible residues prepared from wheat bran by successive treatment with amylolytic and peptide-splitting enzymes. On the other hand, fiber of maize produces relatively little interference. Examination of some 40 wheat fiber preparations yielded a modal value for interference of 36 %, with a high of 78% (18). Uptake of fiber-bound iron was not increased by the presence of substances that inhibited iron binding in vitro, such as ascorbate, cysteine, etc. They, in turn, inhibited uptake of iron independently of fiber, so that the actions of fiber preparations and soluble chelators were additive. Lowering the pH of the solutions to 4.5 or less appeared to permit some uptake of fiber-bound iron, but did not do so consistently. These experiments indicate that complexes of iron with dietary fiber are not easily disrupted by the iron acceptors of either small or large intestine.

Dietary fiber and the oxidative state of dietary iron

It has long been known that non-heme iron is absorbed only as the ferrous form from the intestine. It appears that the presence of dietary fiber preparations favors conversion of iron II to iron III within the range of pH prevailing in the intestinal contents (Reinhold and Garzón, unpublished, 1981). Kojima et al (19) observed considerable oxidation of Fe II to Fe III during solubilization of the iron of cooked pinto bean suspensions by citric acid between pH 4.0 and 7.0 EDTA and other chelating agents acted in a similar manner, and it is possible that the bean fiber may have promoted the conversion. Harris and Aisen (20) have shown that oxidation of iron is facilitated by iron binding agents. Nojeim and Clydesdale (21) report that the conversion of Fe II to Fe III is pH-dependent. Formation of Fe III is favored at pH 6.2 and the reverse at pH 2.7.

The Effect of Dietary Fiber upon Absorption of Iron by Animals

Certain requirements must be fulfilled in order to successfully demonstrate an effect of dietary fiber upon iron availability in monogastric animals: (a) inclusion of enough fiber in the diet to produce the modifications in physiological functions of the gut associated with fiber consumption, e.g. changed motility, fecal volume and weight, water-holding, ion-exchanging behavior and others, (b) limitation of iron intake, (c) observation for a sufficient time to permit the effects of fiber to be manifested, and (d) use of species with a limited capability for destruction of fiber. Lee and Oace (22) question the suitability of the rat in this connection because of the long sojourn of digesta in a capacious cecum and consequent degradation of fiber, particularly xylans. They suggest restraint in extrapolation of findings for rats to other species.

Despite this drawback, a number of studies based almost entirely upon the use of rats have shown that dietary fibers from various sources may impair iron absorption (Table 1). The fiber sources examined most often were fiber-rich mill fractions of wheat, generally bran. The use of isolated fiber components is confined largely to cellulose. Although wheat bran is rich in phytate, the work of Morris and Ellis (34) supported by subsequent publications from the same source, indicates that interference by phytate with iron absorption is not appreciable, and can be disregarded. Liebman and Driskell (35) and Hunter (36) have also found no interference by phytate with iron metabolism, confirming the earlier report of Cowan et al (37). However, Simpson et al (61) very recently recently reported that a phosphate-rich extract of dephytinized bran inhibited iron absorption. Thus, it is not permissible to equate bran with fiber completely.

Among single fiber sources, cellulose decreased iron absorption when fed in sufficient amounts to rats (23,33) but not to monkeys (27) or chickens (31). Agar, carrageenan, alginate and fucoidan decreased iron balance (28) or iron uptake (29) in rats. The difference between the response of iron-depleted and iron-replete rats to alginate is of interest. Iron absorption was decreased in the latter but not in the former (29).

Dietary Fiber and Iron Absorption by Humans

Widdowson and McCance (38) in 1942 measured iron balances of men and women while they ate diets in which wheaten bread of 92% extraction rate or white bread were the principal sources of energy for eight or more weeks. The bread, made of flours of high extraction rate, lowered iron balances despite its higher iron content, although balances did not become negative. Walker et al (39) made a similar comparison of iron balances while white or brown breads were eaten, although at a lower level of intake (estimated to be 30 to 40 % of total energy intake). Iron balances were lowered during each period of brown bread consumption. The authors did not evaluate their findings statistically, however, application of the t test to the data shows the difference in iron balances between the

Table I
The effect of dietary fibers or fiber-rich foods on iron bioavailability in animals.

Authors, year	Ref.	Animal	Fiber source	Criteria	Bioavailability
Stiles et al, 1976	23	Rat	Corn pericarp Cellulose Peanut hulls (7.5 to 30 %, 18 days)	Whole body count	Decreased Decreased No effect
Ranhotra et al, 1979	24	Rat	Cellulose incorp. into bread(10-30%)	Hb repletion	Decreased
Lee et al, 1979	25	Rat	High cellulose bread Bran, soy or veg. flour supplements	Hb repletion	No effect Decreased
Miller, 1979	26	Anemic rat	Wheat shorts (70-210 g/Kg diet)	Hb repletion	No effect
Spiller et al, 1980	27	Pig-tail monkey	Wheat bran Semi-purified corn bran Cellulose Pectin (3,6,9 g/day)	Balance	Decreased
Harmuth-Hoene et al, 1980	28	Rat	Carrageenan Agar Alginate Guar gum Carob bean gum (10% level)	Balance	Decreased Decreased Decreased No effect No effect
Woelbling et al, 1980	29	Rat, Jejunal segment	Alginate Guar gum	^{59}Fe uptake	Decreased Decreased
		Anemic rat	Alginate Guar gum		No effect No effect

Continued on next page.

Table I—continued.

Authors, year	Ref.	Animal	Fiber source	Criteria	Bioavailability
Becker et al, 1980	30	Rat, jejunal segment	Fucoidan	^{59}Fe uptake	Decreased
		Anemic rat	Fucoidan		Decreased
Thompson, Weber, 1981	31	Chick	Wheat bran	Iron in liver, tibia	No effect
			Corn bran		No effect
			Soy bran		No effect
			Oat hulls		No effect
			Cellulose		No effect
			Rice bran (6% level)		Decreased
Harmuth-Hoene et al, 1981	32	Rat	Whole wheat,	Balance	Decreased
			rye breads bran-supplemented		Decreased
Garcia-Lopez, Wyatt, 1981	33	Rat	Cellulose, 5%	Hb repletion	No effect
			Cellulose, 10%		Decreased
			Cellulose, 15%		Decreased
Ranhotra et al	66	Rat	Iranian flatbread	Hb repletion	No effect
Wiemer, Kies	67	Weanling mice	Hemicellulose	Balance	Decreased
Fernandez, Phillips	69	Dog	Lignin	Duodeno-jejunal perfusion	Decreased
			Hemicellulose		Decreased
			Pectin		Small decrease
			Cellulose		No effect
Reinhold et al	18	Rat	Wheat NDF	Uptake, intestinal segments.	Decreased
			Maize NDF		Decreased

periods of white and brown breads to be highly significant. This is contrary to their conclusion that "the retention of iron was virtually the same for low and high phytate diets," the two breads being identified by their phytate contents, (Phytate at the time was considered the major antimetabolite for iron). Cullumbine et al (40) evaluated iron balances while either white or brown rice was being eaten. Although iron retention was lower while brown rice served as the main energy source, the differences were small and not significant. Bjorn-Rasmussen (41) found a remarkably consistent relationship between iron uptake of men and the negative logarithm of the quantity of bran added to the diet.

The foregoing and more recent studies of iron utilization by humans as affected by consumption of dietary fibers or of fiber-rich foods are summarized in Table 2. As with studies of animals, investigations of purified fiber components are few, the main dependence being upon fiber-rich foodstuffs, especially wheat bran as the source of fiber intake enhancement. The composition of the diet used during balance studies may affect the response of iron metabolism to fiber consumption. Thus, diets containing fruits and vegetables in abundance may decrease binding of iron by dietary fiber because of inhibition by ascorbic, citric and other acids present in these foods. Increased absorption of iron would be favored. Such acids have been found to be augmentors of iron absorption (59,61). The unique behavior of iron in the experiments of Kelsay et al (52) in which dietary fiber intakes were elevated by consumption of fruits and vegetables may have its origin in this factor. Only iron among the several bivalent cations studied failed to respond with negative balances. A similar action may have influenced the results of other investigators. Thus, the conventional foods listed by Sandstead et al (50) as forming part of the diet of subjects participating in their balance studies included several sources of ascorbate and citrate. The effects of ascorbic acid and of meat are clearly shown by the experiments of Simpson et al (61). The latter demonstrated that removal of phytate from bran does not diminish its activity in impairing iron absorption by humans. They did, however, find that the

Table II
The effect of dietary fibers of fiber-rich foods on iron bioavailability in humans.

Authors, year	Ref.	Fiber source	Criteria	Bioavailability
Widdowson, McCance 1942	38	Bread, 92% extraction wheat flour	Balance	Decreased
Walker et al, 1948	39	Bread, 95-100% extraction wheat flour	Balance	Decreased (see text)
Cullumbine et al, 1950	40	Brown rice	Balance	No effect
Björn-Rasmussen, 1974	41	Increments of wheat bran in bread	Uptake of radioiron by rbc	Negative correlation r= -0.92
Vellar et al 1968	42	Fortified white vs fortified wholemeal bread	Serum iron	Smaller rise for wholemeal bread
Elwood et al, 1970	43	White vs wholemeal chapattis	Whole body count	Decreased by whole meal
Hoglund 1970	44	Sifted vs unsifted flour	Whole body count	Decreased by unsifted flour
Jenkins et al, 1975	45	Wheat bran, 36	Serum iron	Decreased
Persson et al, 1975	46	Wheat bran	Serum iron	Decreased
Brodribb et al, 1976	47	High fiber diet 6 months	Hematologic	No effect
Sanders et al, 1977	48	Vegans	Serum iron etc.	Normal
Dobbs et al, 1977	49	Wholemeal bread, 100g/day	Whole body count	Decreased
Sandstead et al, 1977	50	Wheat bran Corn bran (26 g/day)	Balance	No effect No effect

Continued on next page.

Table II—continued.

Authors, year	Ref.	Fiber source	Criteria	Bioavailability
Olszon et al 1978	51	High fiber diet	Fecal iron	Neg.correl. with fecal solids(fiber)
Kelsay et al	52	Fruits,vegetables,23.8g NDF/day.	Balance	No effect
Lei et al 1980	53	Pectin 15g/day	Balance	No effect
Monnier et al,1980	14	Pectin	Uptake of radioiron by rbc	Decreased
		Cellulose		No effect
Morris et al 1980	54	Bran muffin	Uptake of radioiron by rbc	Decreased
		Dephytinized bran muffin, 36g bran/day		Decreased
Oski et al 1980	55	Strained pears	Uptake of radioiron by rbc	Decreased
Van Dokkum 1980	56	Increments of bran	Iron excretion	Decreased at high intakes
Faraji et al,1981	57	Bazari*	Balance	Decreased
			Serum iron	Decreased
		Bazari + cellulose,10g	Balance	No effect
			Fecal iron	Increased
			Serum iron	Decreased
Anderson et al,1981	58	Vegetarian diet, 31 % fiber	Hematologic	No effect
Godara et al,1981	59	Cellulose,21g daily	Balance	Decreased
			Serum iron	Decreased
MacPhail et al,1981	60	Wheat bran added to maize porridge with added ferrous sulfate	Absorption of added iron	Eleven-fold decrease
Simpson et al,1981	61	Wheat bran	Uptake of radioiron	Decrease
		Dephytinized wheat bran		Decrease
		Supernate of latter		Decrease

*A fiber-rich Iranian Flat bread supplying about 60% of the enrgy intake during the study.

supernatant solution resulting from dephytinization was somewhat more inhibitory than the fiber-containing residue.

Under less opulent conditions than the preceding American studies, Faraji et al (57) demonstrated adverse effects of high fiber diets in the form of Iranian fiber-rich flat bread upon iron metabolism Elwood et al (43) compared iron absorption from chapattis made from white flour with that from chapattis made from wholemeal flour. Absorption from the latter was lower. Similarly, Dobbs and Baird (49) showed that the percentage or iron absorbed from white bread was considerably higher than that absorbed from wholemeal bread. Serum iron concentrations decreased following ingestion of wheat bran (Jenkins et al,45) or wholemeal bread as compared with white bread (Persson et al,46). Fortified white bread produced a greater rise in serum iron concentrations than did wholemeal bread with a similar level of fortification (Vellar et al, 42).

High fiber diets administered to patients suffering from diverticular disease did not lower hemoglobin concentrations over a six month period (Brodribb and Humphreys, 47). Prolonged consumption of vegetarian diets which are inherently rich in dietary fiber did not impair iron metabolism as judged by hematologic criteria (48,58).

A common baby food, strained pears, inhibited iron absorption in the presence of human milk according to Oski and Landau (55). Although the authors did not attribute the action to dietary fiber, it is a possible suspect.

Use of an intubation technique enabled Matseshe et al. (62) to show that iron introduced directly into the small intestine of human subjects in the presence of cereals was recovered less rapidly and completely than iron from ferrous sulfate or reduced iron in the presence of meat. Bran caused an 11-fold decrease in absorption of iron in the studies of McPhail et al (60). This impairment was not observed when iron was given in the form of Fe(III)EDTA, a response that is compatible with the ability of EDTA to release iron from its combination with dietary fiber.

Examination of the ability of isolated fiber components to interfere with iron absorption has yielded conflicting results. Godara et al. (59) fed 21 g of cellulose daily for 21 days. A significant decrease in iron balance and serum iron concentrations occurred. In the experiments of Faraji et al (57), half as much cellulose failed to produce significant changes in iron balance, although serum iron concentrations fell. There is no agreement, also, concerning the action of pectin. Thus, Monnier et al (14) reported a decreased radioactive iron uptake accompanying pectin ingestion, while Lei et al (53) saw no change in iron balance to be associated with pectin administration.

Estimation of the amount of iron complexed by fiber in cereal-rich diets

The proportion of dietary iron bound by dietary fiber may be estimated by use of the coefficients (13) described in the Section: Affinity of fiber for iron. Such estimates are applicable to the numerous populations that derive major portions of their diets from wheat and maize. Thus, in Central Mexico the median daily consumption of maize has been estimated to provide 14 g of NDF (63). This figure multiplied by 0.30, the coefficient for maize NDF, yields 4.2mg of iron bound by the NDF. With a daily intake of 19 mg of iron in this region of México, the amount complexed is trivial, particularly since consumption of protective foods, including fruits and vegetables, is appreciable. However, in rural Iran, NDF intakes in the form of unleavened flat wheaten breads may exceed 50 g daily. Fifty g multiplied by the coefficient for NDF of wheat, 0.38, gives 19mg of bound iron, a figure that would decrease available iron substantially, although iron intakes in Iran tend to be high (64). However, consumption of protective foods is likely to be low because of geographic, seasonal and economic restraints.

In addition to the complexant action of fiber, it should be recalled that other actions, e.g. changes in the physiological behavior of the gut and increased proliferation of gut flora, may promote losses of iron.

Further studies

Additional measurements of the coefficients of iron binding by dietary fibers from various sources are needed, particularly because the published coefficients are based on single samples of wheat and maize brans. The need is made greater by the finding of Thompson et al (65) that method of fiber preparation affected ion exchange capacity for copper and zinc. It would be helpful to learn if iron is similarly affected. Further studies of the importance of the protein that appears to be an intrinsic component of some dietary fibers in binding of iron and other cations are needed. The extent of binding of ferric iron by dietary fibers needs to be evaluated.

Measurements of iron binding by various dietary fibers in vivo like those done by Fernandez and Phillips (69) using isolated segments of intestine in situ would assist in the appraisal of the extent of interference with iron absorption. Balance studies of larger omnivera also are needed.

Further studies of the effects of dietary fiber from various sources upon iron utilization by human subjects are necessary. Some existing studies are inconclusive because of their short duration; others because of the small samples studied. Long term studies of the fiber-rich, low energy diets of many less developed regions would also be important for evaluation of the iron deficiency that often prevails.

Acknowledgements

I thank my wife, Sally Edwards Reinhold, for help in reviewing the literature and Miss Judith Barba for typing the manuscript.

Addenda

Several relevant studies have appeared since the manuscript was completed. Ranhotra et al.(66) examined the availability of the iron of five types of Iranian flat breads to rats by use of the hemoglobin repletion method. They found no direct relationship to content of fiber (or phytate or protein). Wiemer and Kies (67) observed that the addition of hemicellulose in the form of psyllium to the diets of weanling mice increased iron losses in feces. Fernandez and Phillips (68) measured the binding of iron *in vitro* by lignin, hemicellulose (psyllium mucilage), pectin and alpha cellulose. Affinities for iron of the first two substances were high, that of pectin less, and that of the cellulose negligible. Citrate and EDTA inhibited binding. In further studies made in vivo, lignin and hemicellulose introduced into duodenal jejunal segments of dogs were potent inhibitors of iron absorption. Pectin was less inhibitory and alpha cellulose was ineffective (69).

Literature cited

1. Eastwood,M.A.; Kay,R.M. Am.J.Clin.Nutr.1979,32,364
2. Reinhold,J.G.; Ismail-Beigi,F.; Faraji,B. Nutr. Rep.Int. 1975, 12,75.
3. Ismail-Beigi,F.; Faraji,B.; Reinhold,J.G.Am.J.Clin Nutr. 1977, 30, 1721.
4. Van Soest,P.J. J.Assoc.Off.Anal.Chem. 1963, 46, 825.
5. Robertson,J.B.; Van Soest,P.J. Proc.69th.Meeting Am. Soc. Animal Sci., Madison,Wisconsin, 1977.
6. Van Soest,P.J.; Robertson,J.B. Nutr.Rev. 1977, 35, 12.
7. Cummings,J.H. in Fiber in Human Nutrition. Spiller, G.A.; Amen,R.J., eds. Plenum Press, New York, 1976, p.1.
8. Southgate, D.A.T. in Fiber in Human Nutrition. Spiller,G.A.; Amen,R.J.,eds.Plenum Press, New York, 1976, p.31.
9. Reinhold,J.G.; Nasr,K.; Lahimgarzadeh,A.; Hedayati, H. Lancet 1973, 1, 283.
10. Reinhold,J.G.; Faraji,B.; Abadi,P.; Ismail-Beigi,F. in Trace Elements in Human Health and Disease. Prasad, A.S.,ed. Academic Press, New York, 1976, 1, 163.
11. Reinhold,J.G.; Parsa,A.: Karimian,N.; Hammick,J.W.; Ismail-Beigi,F. J.Nutr. 1974, 105, 976.
12. Camire,A.L.; Clydesdale,F.M. J.Food Sci. 1981, 46, 548.
13. Reinhold,J.G.; Garcia L.,J.S.; Garzón,P. Am.J.Clin. Nutr. 1981, 34, 1384.

14. Monnier, L.; Coletti, C.; Aguirre, L.; Miranze, J. Am. J. Clin. Nutr. 1980, 33, 1225.
15. Mod, R.R.; Ory, R.L.; Morris, N.M.; Normand, F.L. J. Agric. Food Chem. 1981, 29, 449.
16. Thompson, S.A.; Weber, C.W. J. Food Sci. 1979, 44, 752.
17. Reilly, C. Biochem. Soc. Trans. 1979, 9, 202.
18. Reinhold, J.G.; García-L, P.M.; Arias-Amado, L.; Garzón, P. 1982, in Dietary Fiber in Health and Disease. G.V. Vahouny and Kritchevsky, D., eds. Plenum Publ. Co., New York, N.Y. p.117.
19. Kojima, N.; Wallace, O.; Bates, G.W. Am. J. Clin. Nutr. 1981, 34, 1392.
20. Harris, D.C.; Aisen, P. Biochim. Biophys. Acta. 1973, 329, 156.
21. Nojeim, S.J.; Clydesdale, F.M. J. Food Sci. 1981, 46, 606.
22. Lee, B.A.; Oace, S.J. Fed. Proc. 1980, 39, 785.
23. Stiles, L.W.; Rivers, J.M.; Hackler, L.R.; Van Campen, D.R. Fed. Proc. 1976, 35, 744.
24. Ranhotra, G.S.; Lee, C.; Gelroth, J.A. Cereal Chem. 1979, 56, 156.
25. Lee, C.; Gelroth, J.A.; Ranhotra, G.S. Fed. Proc. 1979, 38, 473.
26. Miller, J. Cereal Chem. 1979, 56, 253.
27. Spiller, G.A.; Chernoff, M.C.; Gares, J.E. Nutr. Rep. Int. 1980, 22, 353.
28. Harmuth-Hoene, A.E.; Schelenz, R. J. Nutr. 1980, 110, 1774.
29. Woelbling, R.H.; Becker, G.; Forth, W. Digestion 1980, 20, 403. Chem. Abst. 1980, 93, 230987.
30. Becker, G.; Osterlok.; Schaefer, W.; Forth, W.; Paskins-Hurlburt, A.J.; Tanaka, G.; Skoryna, S.C. Digestion 1981 21, 6. Chem. Abst. 1980, 93, 216024.
31. Thompson, S.A.; Weber, C.W. Poultry Sci. 1981, 60, 840.
32. Harmuth-Hoene, A.E.; Schelenz, R.; Fretzdorff, B.: Rabe, E.; Seibel, W. Getreide, Mehl., Brot. 1981, 35, 65. Chem. Abst. 1981, 94, 190712.
33. García-Lopez, J.S.; Wyatt, J. Private Communication. 1981.
34. Morris, E.R.; Ellis, R. J. Nutr. 1980, 110, 2000
35. Liebman, M.; Driskell, J. Nutr. Rep. Int. 1979, 19, 281.
36. Hunter, J.E. J. Nutr. 1981, 111, 841.
37. Cowan, J.W.; Esfahani, M.; Salji, J.D.; Azzam, S.A. J. Nutr. 1966, 90, 423.

38. Widdowson,E.M.; McCance,R.A. Lancet 1942, 1, 588.
39. Walker,A.R.P.; Fox,F.W.; Irving,J.T. Biochem.J. 1948, 42,452.
40. Cullumbine,H.; Basnayake,V.; Lemottee,J.; Wickramanayake,T.W. Br.J.Nutr.1950, 4, 101.
41. Björn-Rasmussen,E. Nutr.Metab. 1974,16,101.
42. Vellar,O.D.; Borchgrevink,C.; Natvig,H. Acta Med. Scand. 1968, 183, 251.
43. Elwood,P.C., Benjamin,I.T., Fry,F.A.; Eakins,J.O.; Brown,D.A.; de Koch,P.C.; Shah,J.V. Am.J.Clin.Nutr. 1970, 23,1267.
44. Hoglund,S. Acta Med.Scand.Suppl. 1970, 518,1.
45. Jenkins,P.J.A.; Hill,M.S.; Cummings,J.H. Am.J.Clin. Nutr. 1975, 28, 1408.
46. Persson,L.; Raby,K.; Fonns-Bech,P.; Jensen,E. Lancet 1975, 2, 1208.
47. Brodribb,A.J.M.; Humphreys,D.M. Br.Med.J. 1976, 1, 424.
48. Sanders,T.A.B.; Ellis,F.R. Br.Med.J.1977,2,636.
49. Dobbs,R.J.; Baird,I.M. Br.Med.J. 1977,1,1641.
50. Sandstead,H.H.; Muñoz,J.M.; Jacob,R.A.; Klevay,L.M.; Reck,S.J.; Logan,Jr.,G.M.; Dintzis,F.R.; Inglett,G. E.; Shuey,W.C. Am.J.Clin.Nutr. 1978,31,S180.
51. Olzson,E.; Isaksson,B.; Nörrby,A.; Solvell,L. Am.J. Clin.Nutr.1978, 31, 106.
52. Kelsay,J.L.; Behall,K.M.; Prather,E.S. Am.J.Clin. Nutr. 1979, 32, 1876.
53. Lei,K.Y.; Davis,M.W.; Fang,M.M.; Young,L.C. Nutr.Rep. Int. 1980, 22, 459.
54. Morris,E.R.; Simpson,K.M.; Cook,J.D. Am.J.Clin.Nutr. 1980, 33, 941.
55. Oski,F.A.; Landow,S.A. Am.J.Dis.Child. 1980, 134,459.
56. Van Dokkum,W. Ber.Int.Ges.Getreidechem. 1980, 10,207. Chem.Abst.1981, 94, 207584.
57. Faraji,B.; Reinhold,J.G.; Abadi,P. Nutr.Rep.Int. 1981,23,267.
58. Anderson,B.M.; Gibson,E.S.; Sabry,J.H. Am.J.Clin. Nutr. 1981,34,1042.
59. Godara,R.; Kaur,A.P.; Bhat,C.M. Am.J.Clin.Nutr. 1981, 34,1083.
60. MacPhail,A.P.; Bothwell,T.H.; Torrance,J.D.; Derman, D.P.; Beswoda,W.R.; Charlton,R.W.; Mayat,F. Br.J. Nutr. 1981, 45,215.

61. Simpson,K.M.; Morris,E.R.; Cook,J.D. Am.J.Clin.Nutr. 1981, 34, 1469.
62. Matseshe,J.W.; Phillips,S.F.; Malegalada,J.-R.; McCall,J.T. Am.J.Clin.Nutr. 1980, 33, 1946.
63. Reinhold,J.G.; Garcia L., J.S.; Am.J.Clin.Nutr. 1979 32,1326.
64. Haghshenass,M.; Mahloudji,M.; Reinhold,J.G.;Mohamadi, M. Am.J.Clin.Nutr. 1972, 25, 1143.
65. Thompson,S.A.; Weber,C.M.; Berry,J.W. Fed.Proc. 1980 39,785.
66. Ranhotra,G.S.; Gelroth,J.A.; Torrence,F.A.: Bock, M.A.; Winterringer,G.L.; Faridi,H.A.; Finney,P.L. Cereal Chem. 1981, 58, 471. Chem.Abst.1981,95, 167422.
67. Wiemer,K.; Kies,C. Nutr.Rept.Int. 1981 24, 165.
68. Fernandez ,R.; Phillips,S.F. Am.J.Clin.Nutr. 1982, 35,100
69. Fernandez,R.; Phillips,S.F. Am.J.Clin.Nutr. 1982, 35,107

RECEIVED August 13, 1982.

10

Bioavailability of Iron from Bran in Pigs

WENCHE FRØLICH

Norwegian Cereal Institute, P.O. Box 8116, Dep., Oslo 1, Norway

In most countries, cereals are the largest single source of dietary iron. The iron content of white flour is considerably lower than that of whole grain flour and flours of higher extraction rate. In Norway we have no fortification of the white flour, and the contribution of iron from cereals to the diet accounts for only 30%. Our neighbor country Sweden does enrich its white flour, with the result that over 60% of the iron in the diet comes from cereals. The frequency of iron anemia is, nevertheless, the same in the two countries.

Bran has been claimed to reduce iron absorption. The aim of this study was to evaluate the bioavailability of iron in pigs in a diet with a high content of bran (6-10%). The results did not show any sign of inhibitory effect on iron absorption from bran, either in short-term experiments or in long-term experiments. It should be stressed that this applies to pigs and should be tested on humans before any further conclusions are drawn.

Norway is a mountainous country and agriculture is difficult. The result of this is that Norway is importing about 80% of the grain for human consumption. This gives us the benefit of selecting cereals with the quality we consider best, both from a nutritional and technological point of view.

In the Whitebook from the Government to the Parliament called Report No. 32 on Norwegian Nutrition and Food Policy from 1975, (1) the authorities are trying to stimulate the consumer and producer towards a diet which should be suitable. It is necessary to have a diet which provides sufficient energy and which ensures adequate supplies of all necessary nutrients and other desirable ingredients. The nutrition and food policy should coordinate several important objectives and considerations.

0097-6156/82/0203-0163$06.00/0

Objectives of the nutrition and food policy may be summarized as follows:

1. Healthy dietary habits should be encouraged.
2. A nutrition and food policy should be formulated in accordance with the recommendations of the World Food Conference.
3. For reasons connected with the question of supply, the policy should aim at increased production and consumption of food and at sufficiency in the food supply.
4. For regional policy reasons, the highest priority should be placed on utilizing the food production resources in the economically weaker areas.

Considerable shifts have taken place in the number and types of energy-providing foods. The proportion of fats in the energy supply has increased, while the proportion of carbohydrates has decreased with a reduced consumption of starches, although the consumption of sugar increased.

The National Nutrition Council stresses that a reduction of the energy supply from fat and an increase in the energy supply from carbohydrates is desirable. There should be a greater use of starches. An increase in the consumption of cereal products would be a benefit in several nutritional respects.

Over a period of the percent of food consumption represented by grain has gradually fallen to about 70 kg per year per person in 1970. In the past few years, however, this tendency seems to have been reversed and it is today 80 kg per year per person. It is our goal to increase the consumption of grain to 90 kg per person per year during the period before 1990. One way of doing this is to have a relatively cheap and stable price on cereals. Today we have a price system for grain where the price is independent of fluctuations on the world market price and also independent of the producer price for Norwegian food grain.

The extraction rate in Norway of 78-80% must be considered relatively high compared with that of other countries, but even such a flour has significantly less iron than whole wheat flour (Table I).

Table I. Content of Minerals, Vitamin B and Dietary Fiber in 100 g of Different Wheat Products

	Minerals		Vitamin B		
	Calcium (mg)	Iron (mg)	Thiamin (mg)	Riboflavin (mg)	Dietary Fiber (g)
Whole grain wheat flour	40	3.5	0.43	0.15	12.6
Wheat flour 78% extraction rate	20	1.5	0.24	0.06	3.2
Bran of wheat flour	120	12.0	0.70	0.24	52.8

An increase in our extraction rate has been considered. This would result in greater supplies of minerals, vitamins and dietary fiber.

In Norway only 17% of the total flour consumed is whole grain flour. A considerable increase would be desirable from a nutritionist's point of view. The fraction of the flour consumed as white bread has been remarkably stable, although large campaigns have been performed encouraging the use of whole grain flour.

The Iron Situation in Norway

Hemoglobin studies indicate that iron-deficiency anemia is quite common in our population, especially in women between ages 15 and 50.

Cereals and cereal products are not only the largest single source of energy, but also a main source of dietary iron. In many countries the iron content of bread made from white flour is therefore increased by fortifying the white flour with iron. But there is also another way to increase the iron content in the diet and that is to increase the consumption of whole grain flour.

In Norway we have no fortification of flour, a conclusion drawn long after discussions and some years with iron fortification in some areas.

Because of long storage time for flour in Norway, discoloring due to iron fortification has been a result. The added compounds have also been shown to have a negative effect on the storage stability.

For some years the enrichment ingredients were then added to the dough at the time of breadmaking. This turned out to be inconvenient for the bakers, and after a short period, this put an end to the iron fortification in our country.

We in the Norwegian Nutrition Council think it is a better policy to give the consumer information and education about which foods are the best iron sources and to encourage them to eat more of these unrefined products.

Our neighbor country, Sweden, has a different policy. They do enrich their white flour, with the result that 2/3 of the iron in the diet comes from cereals, 42% of the total iron is from fortification. It is worthwhile to mention that the frequency of iron anemia is the same in our two countries.

Common nutritional recommendations are a goal in Scandinavia. Because of the different fortification policies concerning iron, an agreement on iron recommendations has been difficult. With a Norwegian food pattern and with no fortification, it is hard to get more than 15 mg dietary iron per day, which has been the Norwegian recommendation for adult women. The corresponding value in Sweden is 18 mg per day. No agreement has yet been reached, but preliminary steps have been taken. Table II shows current recommendations.

Table II: Recommended Daily Allowances

	Sweden	Norway
Children up to 6 months	10 mg	5 mg
Children from 6 months	15 mg	10 mg
Adults	18 mg	12-18 mg

One way to increase the bioavailability of iron in the diet is to increase the content of factors stimulating its absorption. Ascorbic acid is known to increase the absorption of iron. The Norwegian recommendation of ascorbic acid in the diet was until recently 30 mg per day. But we have accepted the Swedish recommendation of 60 mg per day partly because the bioavailability of the iron could be improved.

Iron and Whole Grain Cereals

An increase in consumption of whole grain flour products is the nutritional aim in Norway. The high content of dietary fiber or factors associated with it, however, present in bran and whole grain flour, may interfere with the bioavailability of iron as indicated by several authors (2,3,4). Phosphate and especially phytic acid present in unrefined cereal products have frequently been said to be potent inhibitors of iron absorption (5,6).

On the other hand, Morris et al. (7) recently pointed out that naturally occuring iron in wheat is predominantly present in the form of monoferric phytate, which (unlike phytate complexed with two or more iron atoms) is soluble at pH 7.0 and above and may therefore be a relatively available form of dietary iron. Conflicting reports in the literature on the effect of phytate on iron absorption might be due to the use of different ferric phytate complexes in the various studies.

Other factors in the whole grain bread have been pointed out as inhibitors of iron. Reinhold et al. (8) concluded that fiber in whole grain products might be responsible for the decreased mineral absorption, because it remains undigested in the small intestine. All these conflicting reports have called into question the value of whole grain bread in the diet.

Bioavailability of Iron from Bran in Pigs

On the basis of this it was of interest to study what influence a high content of fiber would have on the bioavailability of iron in the diet.

For many consumers bran has become almost synonymous with fiber, which is not the case. But bran is the most concentrated form of fiber and cheaply available to the general public. In the work I will present here, wheat bran with a fiber content of 60% was used as a source of fiber.

Previous studies of this kind have in most cases used rats as experimental animals. The high availability of iron in the presence of phytate in rats could be attributed to the presence of an intestinal phytase that might liberate food iron as the phytate is degraded.

It does not seem that the human intestinal tract possesses this enzyme. If phytic acid does influence the iron absorption, a parallel is difficult to draw between rats and humans. As in humans the enzyme has not been demonstrated in pigs and, for this reason, pigs were chosen for experimental animals.

The project was done in cooperation with Dr. Lyso and Professor Homb at the Agricultural High School in Norway. The experiments were started directly after the pigs were born. There were about 10 pigs in each litter, both male and female. The weight of the pigs right after birth was around half a kilo. Right after birth, all the pigs were given an almost iron free diet. In addition to mother's milk they got fodder containing skimmed dry milk, white flour, soya flour, sugar, salt, vitamins and minerals (except for iron). The total content of iron in this diet was 17 mg per kilo. The diet was the same for all pigs, and they were free to eat as much as they wanted until they were taken from their mother, at around 7 weeks old. The surroundings in which the pigs lived were also completely iron free, and because they lived indoors they did not get hold of any earth, in which iron could contribute to the diet. The need for iron in this period is 50 mg/kg diet. After 5 to 7 weeks the pigs became very anemic. The hemoglobin had decreased to around 5 g/100 ml. The normal hemoglobin for pigs is 13 g/100 ml.

At this time the pigs were divided into two groups:

1. The reference group
2. The bran group

The bran group got 6% of bran in their diet. Except for the bran the diet was the same for the two groups. The content of iron in the diets was not plentiful. The total iron concentration was the same in the two groups. This means that the bran group, which had extra iron from bran, had a lower addition of iron in the rest of the diet.

The addition of iron in the reference group was only ferrous sulphate, while in the bran group, 60% of the iron came from bran and 40% from ferrous sulphate.

In this part of the experiment the addition of iron was:

1. Reference group	103 mg Fe per kilo diet
2. Bran group	111 mg Fe per kilo diet

At the time of grouping the pigs were extremely anemic, nearly yellow in color. The growth in this first period was somewhat reduced.

With the addition of iron the picture changed very rapidly. The appetite of the pigs was very good and the growth was for all pigs greater than normal. Also the blood picture altered rapidly, but was different in the two groups.

Blood samples were taken each week for 6 weeks. The hemoglobin and serum iron were determined in each sample. For both hemoglobin and serum iron the values increased most rapidly in the bran group. After 2-3 weeks they had reached a hemoglobin level of 10, while the reference group used a considerably longer time. The same was true for serum iron. This was significant for all the pigs, altogether 10 pigs in each group, with a standard deviation of 5-6%.

The conclusion of this must be that there is no greater risk for iron anemia in pigs with a diet containing a considerable amount of bran and fiber than without bran. Giving the same amount of bran in addition to the diet during a long period, pigs never gave any sign of anemia. On the contrary, there was a tendency towards better iron bioavailability for the bran pigs.

In an additional experiment the pigs were given Fe^{59} to study the bioavailability of iron in the bran diet after continuous bran addition for 8 months. There was no difference in iron in the bran group and the reference group.

Conclusions Concerning Pig Experiment

In these experiments with pigs there were no indications that bran had an inhibitory effect on iron absorption. It seems that iron from bran is as bioavailable as ferrous sulphate even from a diet containing a relatively high portion of bran, in an anemic situation.

This could be expressed in the following way:

1. Iron in bran and whole grain cereal products is as good a source for iron as inorganic iron.
2. Bran does not seem to have any inhibitory effect on the absorption of iron, either on inorganic iron or on naturally occuring iron from cereals.
3. If addition of bran results in a higher absorption of iron, as the tendency is in our experiments, this could be interpreted in the following way:
   a) Iron from cereal products is a better source of iron than inorganic iron.
   b) Factors in bran have a positive effect on the total iron absorption.

It should be stressed that this applies to pigs and should be tested on humans before any further conclusions are drawn.

Experiments on pigs are now being performed where iron from cereals is the only source of iron. So far it seems that the iron absorption is as good for the bran-cereal pigs as for the pigs in the reference group which get all their iron from ferrous sulphate.

In Vitro Experiments on Dietary Fiber

The dietary fiber content of various Norwegian wheat flours (9) with different extraction rates were analyzed. To analyze the dietary fiber content we used a gravimetric method, based on digestion of the samples with pepsin and pancreatin. The method is a modification of the procedure described by Hellendorn et al. and modified by Asp et al (10). The pepsin digestion was carried out at pH 1.5 for 1 hr, and the pancreatin digestion at pH 6.8 for 1 hr.

Insoluble components were recovered by filtration after enzyme digestion, and soluble components after precipitation with alcohol and another filtration.

The fiber values thus obtained were corrected for remaining traces of starch and protein. The ash content of the water-soluble and water-insoluble fiber fractions was determined gravimetrically after ignition at 550°C. (Dietary fiber values do not include this ash).

The water-insoluble fraction constitutes 70-94% of the total dietary fiber, but does not contain measurable amounts of ash. The soluble fiber components, on the other hand, were associated with considerable amounts of ash, and there seems to be a linear correlation between soluble fiber and ash (11) as shown in Figure 1. The nature of the binding is under investigation.

Conclusion

In conclusion, the insoluble fraction, which is by far the main part of cereal dietary fiber, does not bind measurable amounts of ash after digestion with proteolytic and amylolytic enzymes under conditions similar to those in the human gastrointestinal tract. All the binding capacity seems to be due to the small soluble fraction in which the polysaccharides but also most of the phytic acid is recovered.

Thus, if these in vitro experiments reflect what is going on in the intestines, the fibers in bran do not seem to bind ash (including iron), and are therefore in good agreement with the good bioavailability of iron from bran in the pigs.

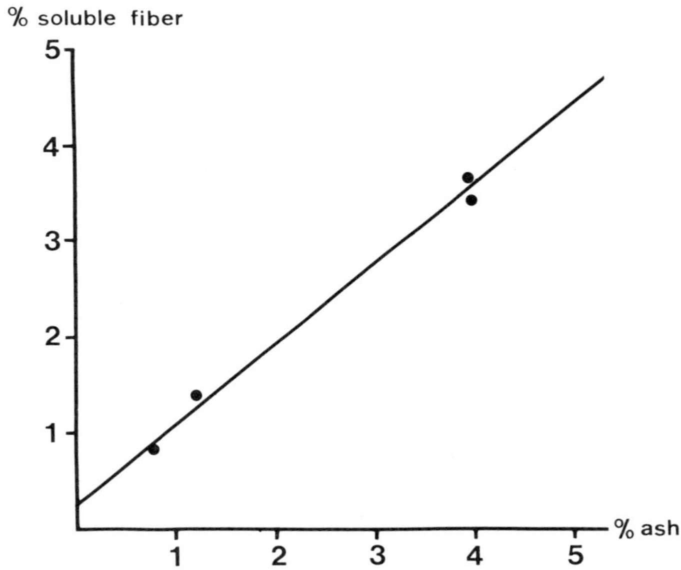

Figure 1. Relation between the soluble dietary fiber fraction and associated ash in wheat products. (Reproduced, with permission, from Ref. 11. Copyright 1980, American Society for Clinical Nutrition.)

Literature Cited

1. Royal Norwegian Ministry of Agriculture: On Norwegian Nutrition and Food Policy. Whitebook No. 32 to the Parliament, Nov., 1975.
2. Jenkins, D.J.A.; Hill, M.S.; Cummings, J.H. Am. J. Clin. Nutr. 1975, 28, 104.
3. Bjorn-Rasmussen, E. Nutr. Metabol. 1974, 16, 101.
4. Widdowsen, E.M., McCance, R.A. Lancet 1942, 1, 588.
5. Sharpe, L.M.; Peacock, W.G.; Cooke, R.; Harris, R.S. J. Nutr. 1950, 41, 433.
6. Hussain, R.; Patwardhan, V.H. Ind. J. Med. Res. 1959, 47, 676.
7. Morris, E.R.; Ellis, R. J. Nutr. 1976, 106, 753.
8. Reinhold, J.G.; Ismail-Beigi, F.; Faradji, B. Nutr. Rep. Int. 1975, 12, 75.
9. Frolich, W.; Asp, N.G. Cereal Chemistry (in press).
10. Asp, N.G.; Johansson, C.G.; Hallmer, H.; Silgestrom, M. J. Food. Agr. Chem. (submitted).
11. Frolich, W.; Asp, N.G., Am. J. Clin. Nutr. 1980, 33, 2397.

RECEIVED August 13, 1982.

11

Bioavailability of Iron and Other Trace Minerals from Human Milk

CHARLES W. WEBER and LINDA A. VAUGHAN[1]

University of Arizona, Department of Nutrition and Food Science, Tucson, AZ 85721

WILLIAM A. STINI

University of Arizona, Department of Anthropology, Tucson, AZ 85721

The iron in human milk is in a chemical form which has a higher degree of availability than either cow's milk or infant formula. The reason for this higher availability has not been determined but theorized to be because of the type of ligand to which the iron is attached. One of the possible ligands discussed was lactoferrin which has a decreasing role of importance as an iron carrier as cited by current research papers. The ligand showing the greatest promise is a low molecular weight ligand to which iron has been found bound in high amounts. The role and/or mechanism of the iron ligand in its absorption is unknown and needs to be further elucidated.

Iron deficiency in infancy remains a common nutritional problem. In infants, milk feeding represents the basis of nutrition and an essential source of iron during infancy. It is felt that iron deficiency becomes a problem after the first four mounths of life. One of the most effective and widespread methods of preventing this deficiency is the use of iron-fortified formulas. The iron levels in iron-fortified formulas are approximately ten times the concentration found in human milk. The controversies concerning human milk versus formulas or cow's milk is the availability of the iron. The iron in human milk is stated to be quite bioavailable, but questions arise concerning the need for iron supplements for infants who are exclusively breast-fed. Further unanswered question or questions is the mechanism involved in human milk which causes it to have a high bioavailability. Some data and theories

[1] Current address: Arizona State University, Department of Home Economics, Tempe, AZ 85281

0097-6156/82/0203-0173$06.00/0

as to how human milk achieves this greater bioavailability are to be presented in the following discussion.

Lactoferrin

Lactoferrin was first identified as a red protein fraction in human milk (1). The milk protein has been called by various names of red milk protein, ekkrinosiderophilin, and lactotransferrin which is in turn very similar in many respects to transferrin, the iron-binding protein of serum. The concentration of lactoferrin in human milk is unusally rich with a range of 7 mg/ml in colostrum to approximately 1 mg/ml in mature milk (2). However, the bovine colostrum contains lactoferrin at concentrations of 5 mg/ml, which drops very rapidly with stage of lactation to where mature bovine milk contains 20-200 µg/ml of lactroferrin (3). Lactoferrin is also found in various other exocrine secretions of the body such as vaginal, nasal, bronchial and intestinal (4-6).

The ability of lactoferrin to inhibit the growth of certain microorganisms "in vitro" has been well documented. The evidence for such activity "in vivo" is not as well defined (7). The role of lactoferrin in antimicrobial activity in the gut will not be discussed in this article.

Lactoferrin's Physical Properties

Lactoferrin has been isolated and identified from a wide variety of animal species. However, most of the studies on structure and iron-binding properties have involved either human or bovine proteins (2). Lactoferrin closely resembles transferrin in molecular weight of 75,000 to 90,000 and consists of a single polypeptide chain that binds two ferric ions. The pI of transferrin is 5.9 while that of lactoferrin is approximately 9.0 (8) and has an even higher association constant for iron-binding. Lactoferrin has the property of retaining its iron even in the presence of a relatively low-affinity iron chelator such as citrate below pH 4.0. Transferrin, on the other hand, looses its iron when the pH is lowered from 6 to 5 (7). There is extensive information in the literature concerning the physical properties of lactoferrin which will not be covered in this paper.

Lactoferrin's Role in Iron Absorption

Infants have a relatively efficient iron absorption of breast milk (9, 10). The close physical properties between lactoferrin and transferrin would suggest that lactoferrin is involved in the transportation as a ligand from the lumen to the intestinal mucosa in a readily absorbed form. Hubbers and Rummel (11) proposed a scheme where alimentary iron binds to a ligand which in turn transfers the ferric ion to a mucosal binding protein which is then transported inside the mucosal cell (Table I).

Table I - Proposed Scheme for Iron Absorption Mechanism.

Lumen			Mucosa		Lamina Propria	
$Lig{+}Fe^{+3}$ ↑↓ [Lig-Fe]	→	binding protein	→ Fe-Ferritin or Fe Transferrin	→	LMW Lig.-Fe^{+3}	Fe Trans-Ferrin

In the case of infants, the ligand may very well be the lactoferrin which transports the ferric ion either to the cell mucosal binding protein or into the mucosal cell directly. Inside the mucosal cell the iron is bound to either transferrin or ferritin for storage. Rat experiments have demonstrated that the absorbed iron passes from intestinal cells to portal plasma largely in a low molecular weight (LMW) form (12). An additional factor would be the age of the infant in which the role of gastric acidity and proteolytic enzyme would have to be considered. As the young infant ages the digestive system develops its ability to function as a complete organ. In neonates, however, iron absorption appears to be less dependent on intermediary iron metabolism and more on the iron supplied by milk.

Lactoferrin's role in iron absorption was demonstrated by the addition of lactoferrin, presumably iron-saturated, to a lactoferrin free simulated human milk. Administered to adults it did not increase iron absorption (13). The addition of apolactoferrin was shown to actually inhibit iron uptake by rat and guinea-pig in everted duodenal sacs, while the addition of Fe^{+2}- lactoferrin had no effect on uptake of iron (14). An additional study demonstrated a negative relationship between duodenal lactoferrin concentration and iron absorption in adults (15). These results would suggest that lactoferrin has no role or even a negative role in iron absorption. Further, additional studies brings into question the role, if any at all, that lactoferrin has in iron absorption. McMillan et al. (13) have shown that the iron in human milk, despite the high lactoferrin content, is more readily absorbed than iron from a simulated human milk of comparable iron content. The addition of lactoferrin to the simulated milk further decreased iron absorption. They further demonstrated that this availability was not affected by boiling the milk which would denature the proteins. A point to consider was the fact that the study was conducted on adults. A second study which demonstrated high bioavailability of breast-milk iron, used the extrinsic tag method and fed the breast-milk to six month old infants (10). Their results suggested that breast milk does contain a factor or factors which actively aid in iron absorption.

The analysis of human milk for the distribution of iron into the various components found iron in three fractions of lipid, low molecular weight form and lactoferrin (16). The total concentration of milk iron varied from 0.26 to 0.73 mg/ml with 15 to 46% of the iron bound to the lipid fraction, and 18 to 50% found in a low molecular weight fraction. Surprisingly, only a small amount of iron was bound to the lactoferrin, which was saturated at 1-4%. These results even further complicate the role of lactoferrin in iron absorption by infants. Further experimental work needs to be done to define the role of lactoferrin in iron absorption, if any at all.

Trace Mineral Cocentrations in Milk

With the exact role of lactoferrin uncertain and the mechanism of iron absorption also unknown, the concentration of iron and other trace elements in human milk is a controversal item. The data involving iron levels in breast milk date from the early fifties to the present time. During the stage of lactation, colostrum, early and mature milk samples are known to decrease in iron concentration with time, see Table II (17,18). The comparison of mature breast milk, 7 days or older, finds a range in iron concentration from 0.21 to 1.28 mg/liter. Weekly, daily and diurinal variation within a given day were demonstrated for iron, copper and zinc in human milk samples (20). Great variations were found within a given day on total yield, fat, and mineral levels (17,20). Table II shows the variation in breast milk concentration for iron and with various claims as to the correct values for human milk iron levels. The differences can be partially explained by sampling techniques, but probably reflect the wide variation found by the different laboratories for iron levels. The maternal diet can affect the iron nutrition during lactation. Lactating rats were fed three levels and the iron status of their pups had a definite relationship to dietary iron levels (27).

Table II. The Average Iron Concentration of Human Milk from Various Sources

Fe mg/liter	Stage of Lactation	Reference
0.40	1st - 5th day	(26)
0.36	5th day	(25)
1.00	1st week	(24)
0.60	3rd week - 2nd month	(23)
0.21	6th - 12th week	(20)
0.86	4th - 6th week	(22)
1.28	2nd - 6th month	(21)
0.49	2nd - 37th week	(18)
0.46	1st - 32nd month	(17)

The breast milk concentration of copper and zinc were found to be just as variable as those demonstrated for iron. Copper-values were demonstrated to range from 0.24 to 1.34 ppm, while zinc was found to range from 5.1 to 1.1 ppm in mature breast milk samples (17, 19, 20). One of the greatest factors in concentration variation was found within the woman herself (17, 20). This diurinal effect was just one of many factors which could lead to the large variation found in trace mineral concentrations of breast milk.

Iron Absorption

Recent studies have demonstrated that iron is better absorbed from human milk than from either cow's milk or formula. Furthermore, that human milk can provide sufficient iron for infants during their first year of life (10, 13, 17, 28). Breast milk and cow's milk are equally poor in iron, containing an average of almost 1 mg/liter. Saarinen's (10) study demonstrated that infants breast fed throughout the first six to seven months of life attained greater iron stores than infants fed a cow's milk formula. The percent absorption of breast milk, cow's milk and formula is given in Table III.

Table III. Percent Iron Absorption From Breast Milk, Cow's Milk and Formula

Reference	% Absorption		
	Breast Milk	Cow's Milk	Formula & Iron
(28)	70	30	10
(13)	15	9	3
(10)	49	19	12
(13, 29, 30)	15-70	9-30	3-12

The absorption values for breast milk range from 15-70%, while cow's milk range from 9-30% and formula + iron average 3-12% absorption (10,13,28-30).

The absorption values were determined under various conditions. In some studies the breast milk samples were tested in adults and not in infants, while another study used an extrinsic tag. The body iron status was determined several ways by measuring either serum ferritin, hemoglobin, serum transferrin saturation and/or serum iron. It was because of these various conditions used to measure the percent iron absorbed that the wide ranges were probably observed. However, the breast milk was always absorbed at a higher level in each particular study examined than was cow's milk or formula. The cow's milk had a higher absorption rate than did the formula + iron (Table III).

Using the data from three different laboratories (17,18,20) the intakes per day were calculated for infants from 1-3 months of age (Table IV). The milk volume of 650 ml was used as an average of several investigator's data (20,31).

Table IV. Trace Mineral Intakes Per Day for 1-3 Month Old Infants Consuming Breast Milk.

Milk Volume/ day	Fe	Cu	Zn	Reference
	mg/day			
650 ml of milk	0.32	0.28	1.04	(17,32)
650 ml of milk	0.27	0.13	1.26	(20)
650 ml of milk	0.23	0.21	0.72	(18)
RDA of milk	10.00	0.30*	3.00	

*suggested daily intake of 0.08 mg/kg/day.

The intake values for iron, copper and zinc were calculated by multiplying the milk concentration values by the volume of milk consumed per day. Interestingly, the data from the three different sources had similar intakes for iron, copper and zinc (Table IV). It should be noted that intakes for all trace elements were below the RDA's given for infants (33). Obviously, the RDA's do not apply to infants who are breast fed but are values to be used for formula fed infants. The greatest disparity is observed for the iron requirement which is 10 mg/day, while breast fed infants have an intake of 0.27 mg/day. The high availability of breast milk iron can account for maintaining iron status in the infant up to six months of age who is exclusively breast fed.

Further calculations were made to determine the mg of iron absorbed per day in infants fed breast milk versus those fed cow's milk and/or formula (Table V). The values were calculated based upon milk intake values for the first through the third month of age. Breast milk furnished a higher absorbed quantity of iron per day than did either cow's milk or formula.

Table V. Mg of Iron Absorbed Per Day from Milk and Formula Sources.

Stage of Lactation	Breast Milk	Cow's Milk	Formula	Formula & Iron
1st month	0.15	0.07	0.03	0.76
2nd month	0.13	0.07	0.04	0.80
3rd month	0.12	0.08	0.04	0.88

The iron fortified formula supplied the greatest available iron to the infant. Interestingly, the total quantity of iron absorbed per day for breast milk decreased from first to third month, while cow's milk, formula and formula + iron increased in absorption. This was caused because the iron concentration of breast milk decreases with stage of lactation. The cow's milk and formula are constant. Their increase in absorbed iron is due to the increase in volume of milk consumed by the infant.

Human milk is a complex, highly variable substance with various factors listed below which can change the concentration of trace elements and possibly the availability of iron. Trace mineral levels were found to decrease with time during lactation. The development of the digestive system of the infant with age will affect potential absorption rate of iron. The absorption mechanism itself is far from being totally understood. The role of lactoferrin in iron absorption is in doubt from the conflicting data available. A different ligand in human milk may be the reason it is so available versus other sources, but at this point in time has not been identified. For these obvious reasons further work is necessary to elucidate why breast milk iron has such a high availability.

Acknowledgements

Arizona Agricultural Experiment Station No. 3547

Literature Cited

1. Sørensen, M.; Sørensen, S.P.L. Ser. Chim. 1939, 23, 55-9.
2. Masson, P.L.; Heremans, J.F. Comp. Biochem. Physiol. (B) 1971, 39, 119-29.
3. Reiter, B. Ann. Reck. Vet. 1978, 9, 205-24.

4. Masson, P.L.; Heremans, J.F.; Dive, C. Clin. Chim. Acta. 1966, 14, 735-9.
5. Masson, P.L., Heremans, J.F.; Schonne, E.; Crabbe, P.A. Protides Biol. Fludies. 1968, 16, 633-8.
6. Masson, P.L.; Heremans, J.F.; Schonne, E. J. Exp. Med. 1969, 130, 643-58
7. Brock, J.H. Arch. Dis. Child. 1980, 55, 417-21
8. Malamud, D.; Drysdale, J.W. Anal. Biochem. 1978, 86, 620-47.
9. McMillan, J.A.; Landaw, S.A.; Oski, F.A. Pediatrics. 1976, 58, 686-91.
10. Saarinen, U.M.; Siimes, M.A.; Dallman, P.R. J. Pediatr. 1977, 91, 36-9.
11. Hubbers, H.; Rummel, W. "Intestinal Permeation"; International Congress Series No. 391, Excerpta Medica: Amsterdam, 1975; p 377.
12. Morgan, E.H. Q. J. Exp. Physiol. 1980, 65, 239-52
13. McMillan, J.A.; Oski, F.A.; Lourie, G.; Tomarelli, R.M.; Landaw, S.A. Pediatrics. 1977, 60, 896-900.
14. DeLacey, P.; Masson, P.L.; Heremans, J.F. Protides Biol. Fluids. 1968, 16, 627-32.
15. DeVet, B.J.C.M.; Van Gool, J. Acta Med. Scand. 1974, 196, 393-402.
16. Fransson, G.B.; Lönnerdal, B.J. Pediatrics. 1980, 96, 380-84.
17. Vaughan, L.A.; Weber, C.W.; Kemberling, S.R. Am. J. Clin. Nutr. 1979, 32, 2301-6.
18. Siimes, M.A.; Vuori, E.; Kuitunen, P. Acta Paediata. Scand. 1979, 68, 29-31.
19. Vuori, E.; Kuitunen, P. Acta Paediatr. Scand. 1979, 68, 33-37.
20. Picciano, M.; Guthrie, H. Am. J. Clin. Nutr. 1976, 29, 242-54.
21. Belavady, B.; Gopalan, C. Indian J. Med. Res. 1959, 47, 234-45
22. Anon. "The Composition of Mature Human Milk"; Report on Health and Social Subjects No. 12. Her Majesty's stationary office: London, Great Britain, 1977.
23. Feuillen, Y.M.; Plumier, M. Acta Paediatr. Scand. 1952, 41, 138-144.
24. Kleinbaum, H. Z. Kinderheilked. 1962, 86, 655-666.
25. Nassi, L.; Poggini, G.; Vecchi, C.; Galvan, P. Minerva. Pediatr. 1974, 26, 832-36.
26. Macy, I.G.; Kelly, H. J. "Milk: The Mammary Gland and its Secretion" Vol II, Academic Press, New York, 1961; p 265.
27. Anaokar, S. G.; Garry, P.J. Am. J. Clin. Nutr. 1981, 34, 1505-12.

28. Saarinen, U. M.; Siimes, M.A. Pediatr. Res. 1979, 13, 143-47.
29. Feuillen, Y.M. Acta Paediatr. 1954, 43, 181-86.
30. Bothwell, T.H.; Finch, C.A. "Iron Metabolism"; Little, Brown & Co.: Boston, 1962; p 114.
31. Jelliffe, D. B.; Jelliffe, E.F.P. Am. J. Clin. Nutr. 1978, 31, 492-515.
32. Vaughan, L.A.; Weber, C.W.; Kemberling, S.R. "Trace elements Metabolism in Man and Animals, TEMA 3"; Arbeitskreis fur Tierer Nahrungsfroschung, Weihenstephan, Freisins-Weinstephan, 1978; p 452.
33. National Academy of Sciences - National Research Council. "Recommended Dietary Allowances"; (9th Ed.): Washington, D.C., 1980; p 125.
34. Stini, W.A.; Weber, C.W.; Kemberling, S.R.; Vaughan, L.A. Studies in Physy. Anthro. 1980, 6, 3-22.

RECEIVED June 2, 1982.

12

Vegetarianism and the Bioavailability of Iron

C. KIES and L. McENDREE

University of Nebraska, Lincoln, NB 68583

Increasing the proportion of plant to animal products in diets should have profound effects on the iron nutritional status of human populations. Such diets tend to be lower in heme iron, higher in fiber, and higher in phytates, all factors which inhibit utilization of iron. In addition, it is thought that vegetarian diets tend to be low in total iron. However, in a laboratory controlled study, vegetarians were found to better utilize iron from a vegetarian diet than were omnivores consuming the same vegetarian diet. These results support the theory that iron absorption is in part mediated by the nutritional needs of the host.

Either because of economic necessity or because of choice based on ethical, health or religious considerations, many Americans are increasing the cereal/vegetable/fruit components of their diets while decreasing the animal product components. The U.S. Dietary Goals would seem to suggest that this is desirable. While the numbers of individuals adopting frank vegetarianism are relatively few, shifts in food intake patterns may result in actual shifts of nutrient intakes or in shifts in nutrient to nutrient enhancer patterns or in nutrient to nutrient inhibitor patterns. By examining nutritional well-being of vegetarians, it may be possible to gain insights on the future nutritional situations of individuals who are merely shifting proportions of basic foods within their diets so as to increase the plant product components and to decrease the animal product components. The ability of plant-oriented diet to provide for adequacy of iron nutrition has been questioned both in terms of total iron provided by these diets and in terms of the availability of iron from plant-based products. This paper will address both of these issues.

0097-6156/82/0203-0183$06.00/0

Factors Affecting Iron Absorption from Vegetarian Diets

In monogastric species iron absorption takes place primarily in the upper small intestine (1). Not all the iron present in foods is absorbed into the body. In the normal adult with adequate stores of iron, usually less than 10% of the iron in foods is absorbed (2). Because of the body's limited capacity to excrete iron, the ability to refrain from absorbing unneeded iron is regulated in the duodenum and is referred to as the mucosal block (1). When the requirement for iron increases as in growth and pregnancy and in various disease and deficiency states, the mucosal block is modified and increased iron absorption occurs. The explanation offered by Underwood (3) is as follows: iron taken into the mucosal cell is converted to ferritin and when the cells become physiologically saturated with ferritin, further absorption is impeded until the iron is released from ferritin and transferred to plasma.

The mechanism of the gut's influence on iron availability is the subject of much controversy. Researchers can be divided into two groups, one holding that the intestine controls the absorption of iron by altering the mucosal avidity for iron, the other holding that the contents of the lumen are changed to make the iron more or less available according to requirement (1).

It is well established that the form of iron in food also affects its availability for absorption. Inorganic forms of iron and iron-protein compounds need to be reduced to the ferrous state and released from conjugation for effective absorption (3). Since most food iron is in the form of ferric (Fe^{+++}) salts, these must be reduced to be efficiently absorbed (2). Similarly, ferrous (Fe^{++}) salts are used preferentially to ferric salts in the treatment of iron deficiencies (1).

There has been much consideration of the efficiency of the absorption of iron from foods of animal and plant origin. Studies in normal individuals on iron absorption from a single food have shown that the mean iron absorption from vegetable foods ranged from 3 to 8% and from animal products from 8 to 16% (4). To determine the effect of vegetable and animal products on iron absorption from ferritin, Layrisse et al. (5) studied iron absorption from ferritin biosynthetically labelled with radioiron in 108 subjects. The administration of this iron compound together with vegetables in a meal resulted in markedly lower levels of absorption than occurred from maize, wheat or soybeans. Iron absorption from ferritin was markedly increased when it was administered with meat, but the absorption from the combination was only about one-half the amount absorbed from meat alone (5). It is difficult to determine the reasons for decreased absorption of vegetable iron sources; however, some researchers speculate that the ferritin administered with vegetable sources is incompletely miscible with a nonheme iron pool or that it actually forms a separate iron pool (3,5).

Many factors have been identified as influencing the absorption of iron. In addition to changes within the host which affect iron absorption and the form of the iron salt, various dietary constituents which may increase or decrease iron bioavailability have also been studied. As diets become more plant product oriented and less iron is provided by animal products, the occurrence of these other dietary factors is also likely to change. Factors which have been implicated include the following: amount of heme iron, ascorbic acid level, dietary protein, dietary phytate, iron-mineral interactions and level of dietary fiber.

Heme iron from hemoglobin and myoglobin is found only in animal flesh products. Considerable research indicates that heme iron is better utilized than is non-heme iron as summarized by Monsen et al. (6). Thus, a shift in diets toward vegetarianism would be expected to decrease the proportion of dietary iron provided by heme, thus decreasing iron availability. Limited evidence exists indicating that not only is heme iron better utilized than is non-heme iron, but that heme iron itself increased utilization of non-heme iron (7-10).

Level of ascorbic acid in the diet has been found to be an important factor in determining non-heme iron absorption (6,10,11). Ascorbic acid intake has been found to be more closely correlated to several biochemical parameters of iron nutritional status than was total iron intake (12). However, timing of consumption is equally important. If non-heme iron absorption is to be increased via this factor, then both the non-heme iron and the ascorbic acid must be consumed at the same time. Considering that important sources of ascorbic acid are all of plant origin, the chances that a shift from more animal-based foods to more plant-based foods will lead to increased consumption of ascorbic acid are good indeed. However, this is not necessarily the case if the shift moves toward a diet based solely, for example, on highly polished cereals.

Phytate-bound iron may or may not constitute available forms of iron to the human as discussed in several other chapters of this book. Earlier work sugests that phytates inhibit iron absorption. Since phytates and oxalates are provided by cereal/plant products, an increase in the plant components of diet is likely to increase the intake of these inhibitors.

Several amino acids are speculated to be effective in increasing iron absorption and can be divided into three categories. These are 1) amino acids which act as buffering agents in the intestine and delay the increase of the pH towards neutrality where iron is oxidized and forms insoluble precipitates; 2) amino acids which form iron-amine chelates that act to enhance iron absorption and; 3) amino acids which act to stimulate iron transport systems within the animal (3). A wide variety of soy products ranging from soy meal to soy protein isolates were found to have a strong inhibitory effect on non-heme iron absorption (13). It is unknown whether the phytate content of these products, the soy protein itself, or some other aspect related to these products is accountable for this effect.

Interactions among minerals affecting their utilization are currently an area of intense investigation. Greger has reviewed impacts of phosphorus and calcium on iron utilization in this book. Interactions of iron with copper and zinc have also been established (14-16). If minerals compete with iron for absorption binding sites, adverse effects on iron bioavailability may occur.

Since dietary fiber is provided only by plant-based products, it is reasonable to suppose that as the animal product components of diets are decreased and the plant product components increase that dietary fiber intake will be proportionally increased. This is, however, dependent upon the kind of plant products which are incorporated. Studies designed to study effects of dietary fiber on iron utilization have given mixed results. Kelsay et al. (17) reported no significant effect of fiber from fruits and vegetables on iron balances of young men. Similar results were reported by Sandstead et al. (18) when wheat bran was the dietary fiber source. Contrary to this, Reinhold et al. (19) found that dephytinized wheat and corn bran had an adverse effect on iron utilization. Results from this laboratory suggest that source of dietary fiber may be an important factor. In our studies, hemicellulose from psyllium and wheat bran inhibited iron absorption, rice bran and cellulose had a lesser effect and no effect was determined when corn bran or pectin were the fiber source used (20-23).

Iron Content of Vegetarian Diets

It has long been known that percent iron absorption is somewhat dependent upon the total amount of iron provided by the diet. Shifts in consumption patterns toward the eating of less red meats may result in actual increases in total iron contents of such dietaries if replacement is made with whole-grain or enriched cereals; however, if the replacement is in terms of milk or cheese, as is often the case with the lacto-vegetarian, the iron consumption may well decrease.

Calculations of iron intake sufficiency have been reported in several papers. Iron intakes of 97 adult omnivores (eaters of both plant and animal products), fish eaters (eaters of plant products but no flesh foods except fish), and vegetarians living in Maine were calculated from 3-day dietary diaries and compared to the 1974 National Research Council Recommended Dietary Allowances (NRC RDA's) for iron (24,25). Intakes of several other nutrients were compared in a similar fashion. Of the male omnivores, fish eaters and vegetarians, 88, 88, and 87%, respectively, had iron intakes which met or exceeded 100% of the NRC

RDA's for men. However, of the female omnivores, fish eaters, or vegetarians, only 4, 36, and 46%, respectively, met or exceeded the NRC RDA's for women; furthermore, 58, 45, and 8% of these three groups failed to consume even two-thirds of the NRC RDA's. These figures suggest that diets of vegetarians were no poorer in total iron content than were those of omnivores and fish eaters and in the case of vegetarian women iron intakes were somewhat better than for the other two groups. Ascorbic acid intake which is known to enhance utilization of non-heme iron was also found to be higher among vegetarian women than for the other two groups studied.

Iron and ascorbic acid intake of adult vegetarian men and women in comparison to the NRC RDA's were also reported by Brown and Bergan (26). Similarly, as in the previously reported study by Tober and Cook, vegetarian men had mean iron intakes of 148% of the NRC RDA's but the figure for vegetarian women was only 62% of this standard. Mean ascorbic acid intakes were 164 and 165% of the standards for adult men and women.

Using a different approach, Abdulla et al. (27) analyzed nutrient contents of 1-day diets of 6 strict Swedish vegetarians (vegans) using a duplicate portion sampling technique. The vegan diets provided 17 ± 6 mg of iron for men and 16 ± 7 mg of iron for women. Iron density of the vegan diets was found to be significantly higher than that for a normal mixed diet (9.0 ± 2.4 vs. 65 ± 1.9). Dietary fiber which has been implicated as an iron absorption inhibitor was also found to be consumed in large amounts in the vegan diets with men consuming 62 ± 9 g/day and women consuming 43 ± 9 g/day. Dietary fiber density was also found to be significantly higher in the vegan diets than in normal mixed diets (29.4 ± 4 vs. 6.3 ± 2).

In a study from this laboratory, iron intakes and iron nutritional status of Seventh Day Adventist students attending Union College in Lincoln, Nebraska were studied. As a beginning study, 28 Seventh-Day Adventist students were asked to keep 3-day dietary diaries. Of the 28 subjects, 15 claimed to be vegetarians and 13 claimed to be omnivores. Most meals and food eaten by the subjects were obtained from the Union College cafeteria which is operated as a lacto-ovo-vegetarian food service. All foods served were sampled for iron analyses. Fasting blood serum samples were drawn on the morning following the taking of the last food recorded. The 13 subjects who claimed to be omnivores actually consumed very little meat during the course of the study; hence, really were much like the omnivores consuming a vegetarian diet.

As shown in Table I, iron intakes of both groups was approximately the same with mean values being only about one-half the NRC RDA allowances for this age/sex group. However, ascorbic acid intake levels were high which might have helped in the utilization of the iron provided. Hemoglobin and hematocrit levels which are sometimes used as indexes of adequate iron

Table I

Iron Nutritional Status of Omnivore and Vegetarian Students Eating a Lacto-Ovo-Vegetarian Food Service Diet (Self-Selected)

	Omnivores	Vegetarians
Number of subjects	13	15
Serum iron (ug/dl)	121	124
Serum ferritin (mg/ml)	36.48	24.84
Hemoglobin (g/dl)	14.05	13.95
Hematocrit (%)	42.04	41.67
Iron intake (mg/day), calculated	10.36	10.60
Ascorbic acid intake (mg/day)	95.6	125

Preliminary data, L. McEndree

nutrition were in the normal range for both groups of subjects as were the serum iron levels. However, the serum ferritin levels of the vegetarian subjects were significantly lower than those for omnivore groups suggesting that the vegetarian subjects had lower iron stores than did the omnivore students.

Iron intakes and nutritional status of 56 older Canadian Seventh-Day Adventist women (mean age 52.9 ± 15.3 years) who had been following vegetarian diets for 19 ± 17 years were reported by Anderson et al. (25). Iron intakes were calculated from 3-day dietary diaries. Mean iron intakes of the 25 vegetarian women who were not taking iron supplements was 12.5 mg/day from food with a range of 7.3 to 19.3 mg/day and mean dietary fiber intake was 30.9 mg/day with a range of 10.6 to 68.3 mg. Percentage contributions of the food groups to total iron intakes were as follows: 32% from bread and cereals, 25% from vegetables, 18% from dried legumes and nuts (including soya products), 18% from fruit, 6% from milk and eggs, and 2% from fats, oils, beverages and alcohol.

Mean hemoglobin, serum iron, total iron binding capacity and serum transferrin levels of the vegetarian women taking iron supplements were 12.9 g/dl, 135 ug/dl, 346 ug/dl and 39%, respectively, and those for women not taking iron supplements were 13.2 g/dl, 107 ug/dl, 312 ug/dl and 36%, respectively. In spite of low iron intakes and high fiber intakes, these vegetarian women exhibited normal biochemical indexes of iron status whether or not they were concurrently consuming iron supplements.

From the results of these studies it would appear that diets of both vegetarian and omnivore women tend to contain less than recommended total amounts of iron. Furthermore, the iron in vegetarian diets tends to come from foods of suspected low iron bioavailability. However, on the basis of biochemical indices of iron status, most seemed to be in adequate nutritional status. Recently, Bergan and Brown (29), reported results of a study involving new vegetarians. Results indicated that 50% had non-acceptable hematocrit levels; 23% had non-acceptable hemoglobin levels, 18% had non-acceptable serum iron levels, 14% had non-acceptable transferrin saturation levels, and 7% had non-acceptable serum ascorbic acid levels.

Comparative Utilization of Iron by Vegetarians and Omnivores

Considerable research exists from laboratory studies indicating that iron contained in vegetarian diets should not be well utilized. Furthermore, results from survey studies suggest that iron intakes of vegetarian women tend to be low in comparison to recommended standards of intake. However, biochemical indexes or iron status among these women do not suggest a high incidence of iron deficiencies. Therefore, a research project was undertaken at the University of Nebraska to study the comparative utilization of iron by vegetarian and omnivore subjects in several laboratory controlled diet studies.

In the first comparison 12 lacto-ovo-vegetarians who participated in several different nutritional studies were pair matched by age, sex, size, weight and ethnic background to 12 omnivore subjects who participated in the same studies. All subjects consumed a laboratory controlled vegetarian diet based on peanut butter, milk, bread, fruits and vegetables for 21 to 28 days. While several different experimental treatments in the form of dietary additives were employed in these studies, only data from the control period when no further experimental variables were employed were used in this comparison.

As shown on Table II, serum iron levels, hemoglobin levels, and hematocrit levels were not significantly different between the two groups. However, the vegetarian subjects did show a significantly higher iron binding capacity in comparison to omnivore subjects (342 ug/dl vs. 312 ug/dl). This suggests that the vegetarians had an increased need for iron and physiologically responded by increasing their capacity for absorption. Fecal iron excretion of the vegetarian subjects was somewhat less at 20.6 mg/day than was the fecal iron excretion for the omnivore subjects (21.8 mg/day) while both groups received the lacto-vegetarian diet. While these differences were only significant at the 10% level of probability, they do suggest trends of biological interest. Percent iron recovery from feces was calculated as the fecal iron divided by the dietary iron x 100. This implies that all fecal iron is unabsorbed dietary iron which is, of course, a false assumption. This calculation is useful, however, in minimizing some of the small variations in individual intakes of iron among subjects. Vegetarians while receiving the lacto-vegetarian diet had a mean fecal iron recovery of 86.37% while the omnivore subjects had a mean fecal iron recovery of 93.2%. This implies (but does not prove) that the vegetarian subjects were better utilizing the iron provided by the vegetarian diet than were the omnivore subjects.

Data from vegetarian and omnivore subjects were specifically examined relative to the experimental plans of several studies which have direct bearing on iron utilization. Six subjects who were participants in a study on effects of several purified fibers on nutrient utilization and who were vegetarians were age, sex, height, weight and ethnic-group matched with six subjects from this series of studies who were omnivores. The laboratory-controlled diet fed to all subjects for 21-28 days was of the lacto-vegetarian type previously described. The basal diet provided 25.3 mg of iron and 14.7 g of fiber. Cellulose, hemicellulose or pectin were added to the basal diet to provide 20 g of fiber/day in separate, randomly arranged periods of 6 to 7 days each.

As shown in Table III, blood serum iron levels varied neither between groups or as a result of fiber supplementation of diets in any consistent fashion. This was also true of hematocrit values

Table II

Iron Nutritional Status of Omnivore and Vegetarian Subjects Consuming Laboratory Controlled, Vegetarian Diets

	Omnivores	Vegetarians
Number of subjects	12	12
Serum iron (ug/dl)	94	95
Iron binding capacity (ug/dl)	312	342
Hemoglobin (g/dl)	13.7	13.6
Hematocrit (%)	42.3	42.1
Dietary iron (mg/day)	23.4	23.4
Fecal iron (mg/day)	21.8	20.2
Iron recovery from feces (%)	93.2	86.3

Table III

Iron Utilization of Omnivore and Vegetarian Human Subjects Fed Laboratory Controlled Vegetarian Diets With and Without Fiber Supplements

Parameter	Mean value while receiving following diet			
	Basal alone	+cellulose	+hemicellulose	+pectin
Blood serum iron (mg/dl)				
Omnivores	96^{a}	95^{a}	94^{a}	96^{a}
Vegetarians	94^{a}	96^{a}	94^{a}	94^{a}
Blood hematocrit (%)				
Omnivores	41.7^{a}	42.3^{a}	42.7^{a}	42.1^{a}
Vegetarians	42.2^{a}	42.4^{a}	42.1^{a}	42.7^{a}
Blood hemoglobin (g/dl)				
Omnivores	13.8^{a}	13.8^{a}	13.7^{a}	13.9^{a}
Vegetarians	13.7^{a}	13.8^{a}	13.5^{a}	13.5^{a}
Iron binding capacity (ug/dl)				
Omnivores	318^{a}	315^{a}	320^{a}	310^{a}
Vegetarians	347^{b}	348^{b}	352^{b}	340^{b}
Fecal iron excretion (mg/day)				
Omnivores	22.4^{a}	22.9^{a}	24.0^{b}	22.6^{a}
Vegetarians	20.3^{a}	20.4^{a}	21.0^{a}	20.3^{a}
Percentage food iron recovered in feces (%)				
Omnivores	88.6^{a}	90.4^{a}	95.0^{a}	89.1^{a}
Vegetarians	80.3^{b}	81.0^{b}	82.4^{b}	80.1^{b}

Note: Values with the same letter superscript not significantly different at $P < 0.05$.

and hemoglobin values. Serum iron binding capacity of vegetarians was higher (significantly so) for the vegetarians than for the omnivores. Both the vegetarians and the omnivores showed some directional changes toward increased iron binding capacity with hemicellulose supplementation and some decreases with pectin supplementation but these changes were not statistically significant.

Fecal iron excretion of the vegetarian subjects tended to be lower than those of the omnivore subjects regardless of kind of dietary fiber variation (Table III). Highest fecal iron loss for both groups was found when hemicellulose was the dietary fiber supplement used. Although similar in direction, the degree of increased iron loss was substantially greater for the omnivore subjects than for the vegetarian subjects. These losses expressed in terms of iron recovery from feces showed a similar relationship. These results again suggest a lesser ability of omnivores than vegetarians to utilize iron from a vegetarian diet and a poorer ability to adjust to the addition of decreased dietary fiber.

Comparative effects of ascorbic acid supplementation of laboratory-controlled diets fed to four omnivore and four vegetarian subjects were investigated. In this case, the diet in the study did employ meat (beef) and fish (tuna). The omnivores continued on the omnivore diet while the vegetarians were given the same laboratory controlled diet but with the beef and tuna replaced with a textured soy product. The iron content of the omnivore diet was slightly higher than that of the vegetarian diet (13.4 mg vs. 12.9 mg). During experimental periods, the basal diet was fed alone or with a 200 mg ascorbic acid supplement.

As shown in Table IV, even though the omnivore subjects continued to receive an omnivore-type diet, these subjects had no significantly better hemoglobin, hematocrit, or blood serum iron levels than did the vegetarian subjects who received the closely matched controlled diet in which meat and fish were replaced by soy products.

Fecal iron losses of the omnivores were still somewhat higher than those of the vegetarian subjects even though the omnivores in this study were actually receiving an omnivore rather than a vegetarian diet. However, it is important to remember that the omnivore diet was also somewhat higher in iron. Hence, in this study the percent iron recovered from feces is a more meaningful comparison. On this basis, the omnivore subjects still showed higher fecal iron recoveries than did the vegetarian subjects suggesting that the omnivores even when receiving the omnivore diet had directionally poorer iron utilization than did the vegetarians receiving the vegetarian diet. Since the omnivore diet contained only 200 g of beef and fish (very low in the typical Nebraska omnivore diet), omnivores were probably receiving a diet more closely similar to a vege-

Table IV

Iron Status of Vegetarians and Omnivores Fed Laboratory Controlled Diets With and Without Ascorbic Acid Supplementation

Parameter	Mean value while receiving following diet	
	Basal alone	+ ascorbic acid
Blood hematocrit (%)		
Omnivores	41.7	42.3
Vegetarians	42.3	42.1
Blood hemoglobin (g/dl)		
Omnivores	13.8	13.8
Vegetarians	13.9	13.8
Blood serum iron (ug/dl)		
Omnivores	119	122
Vegetarians	123	130
Iron binding capacity		
Omnivores	317	318
Vegetarians	329	322
Fecal iron excretion (mg/day)		
Omnivores	12.4	11.9
Vegetarians	11.4	11.1
Percentage food iron recovered in feces (%)		
Omnivores	92.6	88.6
Vegetarians	88.5	86.0

tarian diet than to an omnivore diet. However, the difference in percentage fecal iron recovery was not as pronounced as was observed in the studies reported earlier. In both the case of the omnivores and the case of the vegetarians, ascorbic acid supplementation resulted in trends toward lowered percent fecal iron recovery; hence, assumed fecal iron utilization.

Comparative effects of iron, copper, and zinc supplementation of a laboratory controlled vegetarian diet fed to vegetarian and omnivore subjects was studied in a very limited investigation. In this study, three omnivore and three vegetarian subjects were fed a vegetarian laboratory controlled diet containing defatted extruded soy meal, milk, wheat bread, fruits and vegetables. The basal diet provided 13.5 mg of iron, 2.9 mg of copper, and 10 mg of zinc. During separate, randomly arranged experimental periods, the basal diet was fed alone or plus supplements of of 3 mg of copper or 10 mg of zinc.

As in the earlier discussed studies, no consistent differences were found either between the vegetarian and omnivore subjects or as a result of experimental treatment in hemoglobin or hematocrit levels (Table V). Iron binding capacity of vegetarian subjects were higher than for omnivore subjects but no consistent effects of treatment were observed. The omnivores showed consistently higher losses of fecal iron in comparison to the vegetarian subjects. Both the vegetarian and omnivore subjects tended to have higher fecal iron losses when zinc supplements were given suggesting that iron was being less efficiently utilized. The percentage iron recovery from feces showed similar trends.

These preliminary data suggest that vegetarians may undergo physiological adaptation enabling them to make somewhat better utilization of iron than would be expected from iron bioavailability studies involving the feeding of vegetarian diets to omnivores or involving the testing of particular components characteristic of vegetarian diets with omnivore subjects. This preliminary data, however, also suggests adapted vegetarians response patterns are similar to those of omnivores but that quantitative values differ.

Conclusion

As diets become more plant product oriented and less animal product oriented several factors theoretically should contribute to a decrease in iron nutritional status, particularly, in vulnerable groups such as young women. However, it appears that host adaptative mechanisms come into play which enable individuals consuming plant oriented diets to make better use of these poor iron availability resources than would be expected.

Table V

Iron Status of Omnivore and Vegetarian Subjects Fed a Laboratory Vegetarian Diet Supplemented With Zinc (Zn) or Copper (Cu)

Parameter	Mean values while receiving following		
	Basal alone	+Zn	+Cu
Hemoglobin (mg/dl)			
Omnivores	13.5	13.7	13.6
Vegetarians	13.6	13.6	13.6
Hematocrit (%)			
Omnivores	41.7	40.0	40.5
Vegetarians	42.0	42.9	42.3
Iron binding capacity			
Omnivores	310	322	308
Vegetarians	360	355	350
Fecal iron loss (mg/day)			
Omnivores	12.0	12.5	11.9
Vegetarians	10.4	10.9	10.8
Percentage of food iron recovered from feces			
Omnivores	88.6	92.6	87.9
Vegetarians	76.7	80.7	79.8

Acknowledgments

This work was supported by Nebraska Agricultural Experiment Station Project 91-024 and U.S. Department of Agriculture CSRS W-143. Published as Nebraska Agricultural Experiment Station Journal Series No. 6873.

Literature Cited

1. Crosby, W.H. Am. J. Clin. Nutr. 1968, 21, 1189.
2. Mitchell, H.S., Ryndegren, H.J., Anderson, L. and Dibble, M.V. "Nutrition in Health and Disease"; J.B. Lippincott Co: New York, 1976; p. 47.
3. Underwood, E.J. "Trace Elements in Human and Animal Nutrition"; Academic Press: New York; 1977, p. 13.
4. Layrisse, M., Martinez-Torres, C. and Roche, M. Am. J. Clin. Nutr. 1968, 21, 1175.
5. Layrisse, M., Martinez-Torres, C., Renzy, M. and Leets, I. Blood, 1975, 45, 689.
6. Monsen, E.R., Hallberg, L., Layrisse, M., Hegsted, D.M., Cook, J., Mertz, W., and Finch, C. Am. J. Clin. Nutr. 1978, 31, 134.
7. Hallberg, L., Bjorn-Rasmussen, E., Garby, L., Pleechachinda, R., and Suwanik, R. Am. J. Clin. Nutr. 1978, 31, 1403.
8. Bjorn-Rasmussen, E., and Hallberg, L. Nutr. Metab., 1979, 23, 192.
9. Elwood, P.C., Newton, D., Eakins, J.D., and Brown, D.A. Am. J. Clin. Nutr. 1969, 21, 1162.
10. Cook, J. Fed. Proc. 1977, 36, 2028.
11. Cook, J. and Monsen, E. Am. J. Clin. Nutr. 1977, 30, 235.
12. Bylund, D.M. M.S. Thesis-University of Nebraska, 1979.
13. Cook, J.D., Morck, T.A. and Lynch, S.R. Am. J. Clin. Nutr. 1981, 34, 2622.
14. Lorenz, J.A. M.S. Thesis-University of Nebraska, 1981.
15. Ghani, N.A. M.S. Thesis-University of Nebraska, 1981.
16. Barmann, R.M. M.S. Thesis-University of Nebraska, 1981.
17. Kelsay, J.L., Behall, K.M., and Prather, E.S. Am. J. Clin. Nutr. 1979, 32, 1876.
18. Sandstead, H.H., Klevay, L.M., Jacob, R.A., Munoz, J.M., Logan, G.M., Reck, S.J., Dintizis, F.R., Inglett, G.E. and Shuey, W.C. "Dietary Fibers: Chemistry and Nutrition"; Academic Press: New York; 1979; p. 147.
19. Reinhold, J.G., Garcia, J.S. and Garzon, P. Am. J. Clin. Nutr. 1981, 34, 1384.
20. Wiemer, K., Kies, C. and Fox, H.M. Nutr. Reports Int. 1981, 24, 659.
21. Kies, C. Unpublished data.
22. Kies, C., Fox, H.M. and Vaughan, L. Institute of Food Technologists annual meeting (abstract no. 348), 1979.

23. Kies, C., and Fox, H.M. Am. Assoc. of Cereal Chemists annual meeting (abstract no. 134), 1981.
24. Food and Nutrition Board, National Research Council, National Academy of Sciences, Am. J. Clin. Nutr. 1974, 27, 1095.
25. Taber, L.A.L. and Cook, R.A. J. Am. Dietet. Assoc. 1980, 76, 21.
26. Brown, P.T. and Bergan, J.G. J. Am. Dietet. Assoc. 1975, 67, 455.
27. Abdulla, M., Andersson, J., Asp. N.G., Berthelsen, K., Birked, D., Dencker, J., Johanssen, C.G., Jagerstad, M., Kolar, K., Nair, B.M., Nilsson-Ehle, P., Norden, A., Rassner, S., Akesson, B. and Ockerman, P.A. Am. J. Clin. Nutr. 1981 34, 2464.
28. Anderson, B.M., Gibson, R.S. and Sabry, J.H. Am. J. Clin. Nutr. 1981, 34, 1042.
29. Bergan, J.G., and Brown, P.T. J. Am. Dietet. Assoc. 1980, 76, 151.

RECEIVED June 2, 1982.

INDEX

INDEX

Jacket design by Kathleen Schaner.
Production by Elspeth M. Root.

Elements typeset by Service Composition Co., Baltimore, MD.
Printed and bound by Maple Press Co., York, PA.